THE D

A Journey into a New Life with Multiple Sclerosis

By: Matt Cavallo

This is dedicated to the patients, caregivers, practitioners and lives affected by Multiple Sclerosis.

Published by: Four Horse Enterprises, LLc

For Jocelyn, thank you for standing next to me every step of the way.
For Mason and Colby, one day may this better help you understand who your dad was.
And Ted, thank you for making sure I keep my promise.

Table of Contents

Prologue

I have always known that I am different. From a very young age, I had an awareness of this fact. I could never really pinpoint the how or the why because from the outside I fit my white, middle class ideal. But on the inside I knew that my edges were just a hair too jagged to fit smoothly into the puzzle of my life. In my family, I've always been the stereotypical black sheep. My younger brother is my mother's "BHB," big-handsome-boy, and my sister is the cherished "Baby." I am just Matt and never knew if that was good enough in my parents' eyes. Despite having friends and being a talented athlete, I was constantly searching for validation that I fit in with my peers throughout childhood and adolescence. I shied away from many social situations growing up because I felt misunderstood. Maybe I was ahead of my time. Or behind the times. Whatever it was, my timing was always off. In high school, I wrote and recorded gansta rap way before the Eminems of the world. The only time I felt fully comfortable in my own skin was with my German Shepherds. They were my friends, confidants and sources of pure unconditional love and acceptance. I could tell them anything and they never judged me. As an adult, my insecurities started to take a back seat. I fell in love and married my college sweetheart, Jocelyn, or Joci as I call her, and started a budding career at a real estate development company. Everything in my life was falling into place. That was until one morning when I woke up that would change everything. I was about to find out how different I really was...

Chapter One - Wednesday, May 18

"Come on Zack, keep going boy! You can do it." I sit back on the heels of my rollerblades, holding the leash like a reign as my German Shepherd tirelessly pulls me up the hilly road by my house. It is known as Rollercoaster Road to all of the townies. Nothing is more invigorating than flying down the hill at top speed on my rollerblades but getting up is too much effort without Zack. Zack doesn't mind, though. He would pull me up Mount Everest if I asked him. We must have done this hill thousands of times on our way to walks through the forest.

Zack continues to huff and puff up the hill, never stopping or looking back. He is completely focused on making it to the top. When we finally reach the peak, he looks adoringly at me with his big brown eyes. I gently pat him and say "Good boy."

Now for our favorite part- the downhill run. At the count of three, we take off. Zack gallops gracefully by my side as I let my weight fall forward, gradually picking up the velocity of the rollerblades. The air is clean and crisp on this quintessential New England fall day. The leaves are still clinging to the trees but soon they will cover the ground like a golden quilt. Peeking through the leaves is a bright, almost blinding sun.

Faster, faster. Our momentum builds. The speed and sunshine make it hard to focus ahead but I know we will soon be at the forest entrance at the bottom of the hill. I hear Zack's heavy panting buzzing in my ear but can't see past the white light of the sun....

"It's 6:20. I'm Kevin Karlson, He's Pete McKenzie."

Startled, I open my eyes.

"Stupid alarm clock," I mutter to the empty room.

Five more minutes of sleep. That's all I need. I hate not finishing a good dream. Especially one that involves Zack. *God, I miss that dog.* I try to close my eyes again but it's a futile effort. I can't get back to the dream. I'm up now.

I hear water running, spraying down, splashing lightly. The sound of the shower signals the start of another day. The shades are drawn, but gray light spills in around the edges. Just enough to be annoying.

I try to turn away from the light but my body is stuck in the sheets like I've been dipped in glue. My neck is so stiff that it hurts to fully extend my arms. I roll my head back and forth on the pillow to see if that will help loosen the neck muscles but it doesn't. I drop my head back down on the pillow and squeeze my eyes shut.

Fighting through the stiffness, I raise my head off the pillow and rub behind my ears. My head feels sore and swollen. I ache all over, too. Instead of feeling rested, I feel like I was beaten up in a back alley last night. What the heck happened to me?

I glance over at to Jocelyn's side of the bed. Centered on the night stand is a large reading lamp with a big brass base. The remaining surface of the night stand is littered with empty Poland Spring bottles, Jocelyn's designer reading glasses, the TV remote, and an assortment of magazines. Hidden somewhere in the clutter behind the lamp is the cheap alarm clock ruining my morning.

I need to turn off the alarm, but I am strangely disorientated. I stretch and lunge across the queen-sized bed. It takes every inch of me to find the offending clock radio. I slam the off switch, sending the mess of magazines and bottles crashing to the floor.

"Shit!" I blurt and crash face first onto Jocelyn's pillow.

"You okay?" Jocelyn calls from bathroom. Her shower has stopped. "What's all the commotion in there?"

"Nothing … I'm fine!" I holler back as I try to pull

myself together. After living with me for the past six years, my ever-patient wife is accustomed to my absent-minded, accident-prone ways. I turn my focus on the scene of the crime. Hopefully those water bottles weren't full. I'd hate to ruin Jocelyn's *People Magazine* before she reads about the latest celebrity break-up.

I try to crawl across the bed but can't free my legs from the sheets. My legs feel like they're both wrapped with hundred pound weights. It takes great strength to drag each leg out of each fold in the sheets. I get the top half of my body to the edge of the mattress and reach down. The water bottles are still just out of reach.

I stretch out as far as I can until I have to catch myself with my hands and arms to keep from nose diving into the floor. My T-shirt falls down around my neck and face now as I began picking the trash off the floor with one hand while supporting myself with the other.

The lights come on.

"Oh, that's real attractive!" My wife sarcastically laughs as she looks at my half-naked body hanging half off the bed.

"Admit it," I reply. "I've got a great ass!"

"That was the main reason that I married you!" She laughs again. "Sooo ... what happened in here, exactly?"

"Never mind that now. Joci, I'm stuck here. Come help me up."

My head is so close to the floor by now that my hair could be a mop. I watch Jocelyn's perfectly manicured toes as she snakes her way through the furniture in our cozy bedroom. The old floorboards creak as she comes toward me, twisting to squeeze in between the bed and TV cabinet, which is only inches past the foot of the bed.

Finally, she's standing in front of me. Even upside down, she's hot. She's often mistaken for Kirsten Dunst, though, she hates the comparison. Right now, her blonde hair is pulled back in a shower-soaked pony tail and her slender body is wrapped provocatively from breast to thigh in a purple bath towel. There's not much left to the imagination. Not that mine needs much.

"Matty! Now how did you manage to get yourself into this mess?"

She squints her eyes like Mr. Magoo as she tries to ascertain how I ended up in such a predicament. She's nearly blind without her glasses or contacts. She mostly wears contacts, except when she gets up in the morning or right before bed.

"Well," I reply, "I was trying to turn off the alarm when I kind of knocked everything over. Next thing you know, I sort of slid off the bed trying to clean up."

I squirm and push myself up from the floor, but I'm too far over the edge of the bed to get back up.

I bat my eyes at her. "Ma'am, would you kindly help me up?"

She rolls her eyes and shakes her head.

"Only you," she laughs. "I'll grab your feet and pull you back up." She walks back around the bed.

"Okay, careful now," I say as she disappears behind me. "I'm two hundred pounds of man here, Joci. Let's try not to throw your back out, okay?"

She laughs. "Don't act like this is the first time I've picked you up off the floor, Matt."

I grimace. "Touché."

Next thing you know I am being pulled up from my feet. I think. I mean I feel the friction of my body being pulled across the sheets, but I don't feel her hands against the skin of my legs. I only have the sensation of pins and needles in my legs and my neck is still stiff, too.

Back up on the bed, I roll over and look up at my wife, who is smiling down on me. She drops the purple towel and begins to dry off. I wriggle over to my side of the bed to get a better look. She slowly traces the curves of her body with the towel, massaging her wonderful breasts in the process.

"Don't you have to get ready for work?" she asks

"In a minute...."

I swallow the frog in my throat. I'm suddenly feeling a tingling sensation starting in my chest and spreading down my torso. My mind instantly shifts gears as I shrug off the strange sensations. Plus, work can wait.

She lifts one leg on the bed and bends forward toward me, delicately drying her inner thigh. Then she turns and dries her lower back, completely oblivious to the fact that I am instantly aroused. So much so that I reach down into my boxers to give myself a little head start. This has to be quick. Jocelyn takes her job seriously. I'll have to—

Umm ... wait. Something's not right here.

I look down to see that despite my arousal I don't have an erection. I am more than a little unsettled at this point. I feel a hot rush of panic in my chest. This has never happened to me before. Does this ever happen to a guy at the ripe old age of twenty-eight?

"You okay over there? You look like you saw a ghost or something." Jocelyn asks.

"I'm fine, just...um not feeling that great. I think I tweaked my back last night in my sleep somehow. A shower should help."

"Need me to get you anything."

"No. Just help me up."

"Ok," she says as I'm finally able to swing my heavy legs over the side of the bed. She reaches down and helps pull me up. I wobble weak on my legs and feel a bit dizzy. My whole body is in some sort of fog that I just can't shake. I start to lose my balance and reach out to catch myself with a hand against the wall.

"Seriously, are you okay?" Jocelyn looks more concerned now. "You really don't seem like yourself this morning."

Trying to minimize the situation, I say, "Yeah, you know just need to wake the body up and get those juices flowing."

She raises her eyebrows, not convinced by my lame attempt at humor but decides not to press further. "Just please be careful. You probably overdid it at the gym yesterday." She glances at the clock and quickly turns towards the closet to continue getting ready. "Oh, I've gotta hurry. I'm running late."

With Jocelyn focusing on her wardrobe choices, I start my journey to the bathroom. The bottoms of my feet are numb and the pins and needles sensation seems to have spread all the way up my legs. Since I can't feel the floor under my feet, I slowly wobble down the hallway using the walls as crutches.

Once inside our small bathroom, I quietly close the door behind me, then face myself in the mirror. My dirt-brown hair sits like a helmet on my head, and my pale skin attests to the sun's long winter absence in these here parts. My raccoon eyes are sunken into my head. What the hell is going on with me today? This is the weirdest thing that has ever happened to me. I am completely perplexed right now as to why my legs won't work. Did I overdo it at the gym yesterday? No, not that I remember. There has got to be some logical explanation for all of this. I bet I'll be fine after a nice hot shower. *Deep breath. No need to panic.*

"You got to take better care of yourself," I tell the man in the mirror.

"What?" Jocelyn calls from the bedroom. "Did you say something?"

"No. Nothing. I was just talking to myself."

Our bathroom is small with powder blue walls, white fixtures and a window that looks out to the street when the blinds are open. There is one sink with a toilet next to it. Across from the toilet and sink is the tub.

I move left of the sink and position myself in front of the toilet, place my left hand on the wall in front of me so I don't fall down. Most mornings I would be wrestling my morning hard-on like an out-of-control fire hose to keep from spraying everything but the bowl. Today, however, my penis is hanging limp and shrunken, like I just got out of the pool. As I stare into the toilet bowl trying to comprehend my current state of impotency, I realize things are much, much worse than I thought. I can't pee! I feel my chest start to tighten up again in panic. How is this possible? I want to scream but I can't get any words out.

I move, change my position, move again, still holding myself upright with a hand on the wall. I lean closer to the toilet.

NOTHING!!

I shift my weight again, reposition my legs, and change my distance from the bowl.

Still NOTHING!

A knock on the bathroom door startles me.

"Matty! I need to get in there. I need to dry my hair. I'm late!"

"One minute."

I can't let her see me like this. How would I explain this to her? Jocelyn is the worrying type. I am not even sure what is going on so I don't want freak people out for no reason. There has to be a simple explanation for all of this. I just haven't figures it out yet. I need some time to think. What to do? What to do? My brain is racing. My heart is pounding. No place to hide but the shower. Ah, a brilliant idea. Pee in the shower. She'll be none the wiser.

"Can I come in, please?" She begs.

"Sure."

Just as she opens the door, I flush the toilet to create the illusion of successful urination. She comes in, stands at the sink, and pulls the hairdryer out of the drawer making our small bathroom really crowed. I try to twist around behind her and reach into the shower to get the water going. Luckily, I get the shower going without falling flat on my face.

The pins and needles in my feet persist. I look down at the floor. Bare tile. Jocelyn must be washing the bathmats. But shouldn't the tile be cold? If it's cold, I sure can't feel it. I wish I could feel something, anything.

I strip down, pull the shower curtain back, and carefully step into the tub. Jocelyn is too distracted by her hair drying to notice my awkward shower entry. I grab the shampoo and lather up.

God, I really have to pee. It's starting to consume me. I can't think about anything else. The hair dryer's still running so I decide to take a chance. I lean against the wall and push hard from my gut, hoping to see the golden stream.

Still nothing.

I hear Jocelyn turn off the hair dryer, put it away, and leave the bathroom. The shower is really steaming. The steam feels good in my lungs, but it is stinging my legs and hurting like hell. The pain is becoming unbearable.

Jocelyn returns to the bathroom, pulls back the shower curtain, and leans forward for a good-bye kiss.

"I love you." She says and kisses me, "Have a good day. See you at the gym after work."

In the interest of acting normal, I force a smile and utter, "Love you, too."

She quickly exits the bathroom and closes the door behind her. I wait a minute and then cut the shower. Carefully, I pull myself out of the shower, grab the towel off the sink, and dry off. After a quick shave, I manage to waddle back down the hall to the bedroom, still using the walls to hold myself up.

I enter our bedroom just in time to hear the weather report on the news. Great, heavy rain and low 50's. On any other given day I would be worried about how the weather is going to affect my commute but at this moment I just want to perform a simple bodily function. Confused and naked, I stare blankly at the TV trying to figure out my next move.

Suddenly without warning, my bladder is about to explode. I have to do something, and quick. I labor back into the bathroom with a temporary burst of strength and — desperate measure — pull down my pants and sit on the toilet. I strain. I clench my stomach. Pushing and pulling.

Is there such a thing as urination constipation?

I'm about to cry from frustration and pain when I hear drops hitting the water. Sporadic at first, followed by a steady stream. Then sporadic. Then a steady stream. Then drop, drop, drop. Then a steady stream. I feel like Austin Powers being thawed out after twenty years on ice and, God, it feels good to empty my bladder. Wait a minute. I spread my legs and look down into the toilet. I can see the golden stream, but there's no sensation of it leaving my body. Not only are my legs and feet asleep, but my penis is too. How is that even possible?

This is all way too much for me to deal with right now. I convince myself that it will get better as the day goes on. Since I don't feel sick, I decide that I need to go to work. I've played sports my whole life and I've had to play through injuries, so this is nothing new for me.

I lurch out of the bathroom and back to the bedroom. Not caring what I look like today, I grab a pair of boxers and the closest polo shirt and khakis from the closet. Sitting on the bed, I awkwardly dress myself. Next socks and shoes. I wrestle with my numb feet trying to squeeze them into socks and shoes that now seem two sizes too small. Why don't I have any slip-on work shoes? These shoelaces are getting the best of me! Never one to give up, I am finally fully dressed and ready for work. I muster up what little energy I have left to make my way to the kitchen, take my lunch out of the refrigerator and head outside. Once outside of our small mid

'50s ranch, I face the five brick steps that lead to the driveway. How do I walk down steps when I can't feel my feet?

"Here goes nothing" I think to myself. Deep breath. I tightly grip the cast-iron railing and set forth. I drop my left foot blindly onto the first step. I cannot feel my shoe hit the brick step below, so I grab the railing tighter and then bring my right foot down hesitantly. Typically, I could jump down these steps, now seemingly overnight my ability to walk has dramatically deteriorated

Cautiously, I make it to the bottom of the five steps and look back up to the house. Mentally and physically these five little steps seem like Mount Everest. I have no business leaving the house in this condition. I let out a heavy sigh. I can't go back up those steps right now, though, either. This is going to be a long day but I convince myself that it HAS to get better soon.

Chapter Two - Not So Typical Morning Commute

I stand next to my white Ford Ranger and look out at the busy street. We live at the bottom of a cut-through street, and normally each day it is a struggle to pull out of the driveway with all the traffic. Today, it will be a miracle to get out alive since I have no sensation in my lower body.

I look up at the heavy pewter sky. The morning rain has let up a bit, though not much. The slick roads are definitely going to be a factor in my commute. It is cold, too. The calendar may say it is spring is here, but winter has not yet called it quits. It is more like what you would expect in late February or maybe early April in Massachusetts, definitely not the end of May.

I can't remember the last time I saw the sun. I've been so damned irritable and fatigued for the past couple of months and know that the weather is partly to blame. Maybe I have Seasonal Affective Disorder, but more and more I have been missing Arizona. A little over a year ago when I graduated from Arizona State University, I convinced Jocelyn that we should relocate here to the greater Boston area, on the South Shore where I grew up and my parents still live. Now, I'm having second thoughts. Maybe it's true what they say, you can't go home again.

I yank open the truck door and, using mostly upper-body strength, pull myself and my dangling legs inside the door. My truck is nothing flashy and about as basic as you can get. No power windows, locks, or mirrors. Standard transmission. But the lease is up in November, and with it a lifetime of bad car loans. The inside is littered with empty coffee cups and fast food bags and then there is the fragrance derived from a mixture of dust, smoke and vanilla air freshener.

I should probably take better care of it, but we are planning on turning the truck in at the end of the lease, which makes me kind of sad. I have had some great adventures and many memories attached to this truck. But mostly when I think of the truck, it makes me think of Jocelyn. I had been dating Jocelyn for about three months when my Jeep died, leaving me without a car or way to get to work. The only car that I could finance was this plain Ford Ranger and even still I needed to come up with a down payment. Without even asking and with no expectations of repayment, Jocelyn offered to give me the money. I've never told her, but it was right then that I knew I was going to marry her. It might seem odd, but I knew that if she was willing to take that big a risk on me, then she really loved me for the person I am.

Before starting up the engine, I take a deep breath and adjust the rearview mirror to look at myself again. My eyes are tired and heavy in the sockets. I look like I have a fever, but still don't feel sick. Maybe I was bitten by a vampire in my sleep. Only something that bizarre could explain these strange symptoms.

Then something else occurs to me: how am I going to operate the brake, clutch and gas if my legs and feet don't work? Testing my numb legs, I press the clutch and brake pedals down. I bend and look to see if my feet are even on the pedals. They are. Left on clutch, right on brake. I watch myself move my right foot to the gas pedal. There is a slight, rubber-squeaking, popping sound in the gas-to-brake exchange. If I keep the radio off during the drive, maybe I can key in on that sound to know my feet are actually on the pedals.

I test further. I lift my right foot and move it to the left. Again there is that rubber pop. It is subtle, but I hope it is loud enough to let me concentrate on the road and be confident that my feet are where they are supposed to be. I am also encouraged to find that I have enough muscle control to push down and release the pedals. But I don't know how much resistance the pedal provides.

I shake the gear stick in my hand, take another deep breath, and look at myself again in the rearview mirror.

"Ninety percent of life is just showing up," I say out loud.

Twisting the key in the ignition, the engine springs to life. I depress the clutch, release the emergency brake, and roll down to the bottom of my driveway. After a minute, a good Samaritan lets me out into the traffic stream. Since my driveway is on an incline, I am able to roll backwards into the traffic lane. I cut the wheel left, and then press the clutch and brake to switch from reverse to first.

The gears grind as I jam the stick into first. The truck lunges forward, almost hitting the car in front of me.

"SHIT."

I hit the brake hard. My body jerks. I catch my body just short of the wheel and a shock wave of anxiety surges through me. I look back up the driveway.

Stay home, you idiot! How can you possibly work the clutch with no sensation in your legs? Squeaks and pops? Get real. Go back inside. Call the doctor. Crash on the couch and play video games. Work will understand!!

"Even if I call in sick," I tell myself out loud, "I'll need a coffee."

Why am I talking to myself today? Have I lost my mind along with control of my lower body?

Dunkin' Donuts is less than a mile down the street to the right, going the opposite way of traffic. The drive will be a good way to see if I can actually make it without killing myself. Or someone else.

I roll to the stop sign at the bottom of our street and head south to Dunkin' Donuts. As I drive, I feel like I am in a sit-down arcade driving video game. The Ranger's pedals don't seem real. It is like I am floating- not connected to the truck in any way. At least having a numb lower half absorbs all the bumps on this pothole filled road. A small silver lining moment.

I pull into the Dunkin' Donuts drive-thru and order the usual large regular coffee, which in Dunkin'-Speak is coffee with two creams and three sugars. After getting my coffee and my change, I pause at the exit to the street. Two paths diverge on a paved road. If I go right I can go home, take it easy, and talk to the doctor about this strange occurrence of complete numbness from the waist down. To the left is the promise of traffic, trains, and another day at the grindstone.

"Well," I tell myself, "I've made it this far."

I take another chug of coffee. I don't want to go to the doctor yet. This has only been going on for a few hours. It is bound to improve soon. Why waste a sick day? I come from a long line of stubborn Italian males who only use sick days for what they are truly intended for: golf and hangovers. Plus, what is a doctor going to do? I doubt there is a magical pill for numbness.

Traffic barely inches along as I wind down the highway onramp. It never ceases to amaze me. We have crappy weather here at least half the year and yet if the roads are even slightly damp everyone forgets how to drive.

The stop-and-go motion of the drive coupled with my intense concentration on the pedals and shifting starts to get the best of me. That panicky feeling begins in my chest. Then pressure in my lungs and throat. Butterflies in my stomach. Irritability in every fiber of my being. There is only one cure for this anxiety. I reach under the driver's seat and fumble around, searching for my Marlboro Lights.

I am a closet smoker. I hide it from my wife, my work and my family. Not that I care if they know I smoke, I just don't want to have to hear the constant nagging about quitting. I get it. Smoking is bad for you but I've been hiding it for as long as I can remember. When I was a teenager, I used to try to hide it from my parents. It was almost like a game. I carried a kit of cologne and gum with me at all times. I think they still knew, but my Mom never said or did anything about it other than leaving the occasional article about the dangers of smoking under my door. Dad just wanted to avoid the confrontation. Now, here I am an adult and I'm recreating those childhood mind games in my marriage.

Since I only smoke when I am alone, I use the time between my daily interactions with people to smoke as many cigarettes as humanly possible. It's my daily routine, a mathematical game, if you will. If I smoke five cigarettes before I get to work, then I can work the day without a smoke break. People around the office don't know I smoke, so I don't wear the invisible badge that says, Matt Cavallo, Office Smoker.

By my second cigarette, traffic is at a standstill. My legs and feet are still noticeably absent as I maneuver the clutch, methodically listening for the squeaking rubber and the pops, which are harder to hear over the engine and road noise than I had hoped before I left the house. I still can't gage the pressure I am applying to the pedals, which results in violent jerks every time I shift. This cause-and-effect action is sending my anxiety level off the charts. Good thing I have plenty of cigarettes.

Plus, I am in no rush to get to the train today. I hate the train. Rush hour on the highway is nothing compared to being squeezed into those little subway cars where you're on top of each other like lobsters in a grocer's tank. Breathing germ-filled, stale air while fighting for elbow room or even to have both feet planted squarely on the floor. Without fail, there's always someone near you who's coughing or feels that deodorant is optional. But I can't afford to park in Boston five days a week. Hell I can barely afford to catch the train near my house five days a week.

Between my house and the North Quincy T station there are four train stations. I pass them all along the way. With my hatred of the train, I have my reasons for making the drive to North Quincy, the biggest one being money. Jocelyn controls our finances and believe me, it is better that way. She gives me a weekly allowance. By driving to North Quincy Station, I save $4.25 daily in parking and train tokens. Right now, every dollar counts. Especially with the price of cigarettes being a ridiculous $5.25 a pack. Oh, and the little fact that Jocelyn has no clue that I buy a pack a day.

I fire up another cigarette as I wind through Hancock Street in Quincy. Hancock Street is a tight, hilly, two-lane road. It demands that you work the clutch and shift gears constantly, making it about the worst possible place for me to be driving right now. I roll past Quincy Center Station.

"I should just pay to park," I say out loud. I don't need to save money today. I have a full pack of smokes.

I fire up another smoke as I pull past Wollaston Station. Stopping here will only set me back three bucks. All I would need to pay for is parking, not an additional token. But three bucks is three bucks. And I can't exactly ask Jocelyn for three extra bucks for smokes. Maybe if people would stop educating me on obvious health concerns. Maybe if people could accept me as a smoker instead of passing judgment. Maybe if the stars were aligned in a certain way…. Maybe I'm just a guy with a million excuses. Maybe one of these days I'll be completely honest with myself and admit that I'm a smoker. Maybe.

By the time I finish obsessing about paying for parking at Wollaston, I am pulling into my usual train station, North Quincy. My obsessing has led to me paying the three bucks to park. For an extra buck and quarter, I could have just parked at the Braintree station, saved myself a half an hour on the road, and been guaranteed a seat. *Real nice, genius.*

The overcrowded subway train rattles slowly along the rails. I have the good fortune of being the last one to board the train, so I am wedged up against the door. That gives my limp legs some support. I look out the windows on the other side of the crowded train toward the Marina Bay skyline.

Rush hour on the train, morning or evening, can be deeply depressing. I think the weather has everyone down because this morning, with the amount of people on the train, it seems especially quiet. Everyone is silent, obeying the unspoken code of the morning commute. We march off soundlessly to be chained to our desks, where we'll spend the day gazing out windows (if our offices have windows) and dreaming of what could have been.

Stop after stop I maintain my post, leaning on the door. I really want to ask someone to sit down before I fall down, but what can I say? "Hello, my name is Matt. My feet, legs, and penis are numb. May I please have your seat so I don't fall down?" They'd probably call the cops.

Then it occurs to me: there is no way I can exit at my usual stop today. I usually disembark at South Station, which is over a mile walk to my office. Typically I enjoy the walk because it allows for a couple of smokes before the work day. I know the subway system by heart, so I know there is a stop closer to my office. The only problem is that stop requires transfers to two additional trains. I could spend ten bucks and take a cab from South Station but there is no way I'm doing that. I need to make a quick decision. Completely confused, I freeze as the train stops at my usual exit. *Guess I am going to attempt the train transfers.*

"Next stop, Downtown Crossing. Change here for Orange Line."

The train pulls to a stop, and the momentum of the exiting passengers carries me safely to the platform. I wobble my way down the dirty, white-tiled corridors of Downtown Crossing Station. People push me aside as they rush by, but I remain composed and continue like a blind man, my right arm on the wall, my left arm extended, palm at waist. My legs are extremely heavy. I still do not feel anything- other than exhaustion that is. I am so focused on just making it to the office, though, that I give little thought to the numbness.

I arrive at the platform just in time to board the outbound Orange Line train. Miraculously, I spot an open seat. When I sit down, however, the pins and needles seem to intensify. I bury my head in my hands and try to catch my breath. This is more stressful than I could have imagined. The intercom beeps again immediately.

"Next stop, State. Change here for the Blue Line."

I pull myself up, using the hand-rail pole, and wobble my way down the huge, filthy State Street Station corridor. It is like I am walking in concrete shoes. Each step drains me of precious energy. No doubt that a smoke break will recharge my battery, but there's no smoking down here in the bowels of the subway system.

I board my last train. With only one stop left, I do not bother looking for a seat. I just lean against the door, exhausted. The intercom beeps again.

"Next stop Aquarium."

I pour myself out of the train and onto the platform. This subterranean train station is meticulously clean. For the tourists, no doubt. Its cavernous, concrete walls are adorned with life-size posters of the New England Aquarium. Seals, giant sea turtles, penguins and leaping dolphins all frolic in the sky blue water.

The posters remind me of a TV commercial that used to air between *The Brady Bunch* and *The Monkees'* reruns when I was a kid in the early 1980s. It was about a family with a boy and a girl who are spending a happy day at the Aquarium. The kids are in awe of the fish, screeching out, "Wow!" and "Neato!" at every turn. Then the little girl starts flailing her arms and kicking her legs in an uncoordinated waddle and yells, "I caan waalk like a penguin!" As first-graders, my friends and I would over exaggerate the little girl's walk on the playground at recess and yell in our most obnoxious voices, "I caan waalk like a penguin!"

I chuckle to myself as I get on the escalator. *I caan waalk like a penguin!*

The air is crisp as I exit the escalator on the red brick sidewalk of lower State Street. There is a strong smell of urine in the air. This is a hot spot for the homeless at night, but it's also the corner where the tourists can catch horse and carriage rides around the city in the evening. The uneven brick sidewalks are not a big help to my shuffling feet, but I try to do my best impression of a regular guy walking down the street. My slow, uncertain steps draw obvious stares from passersby.

I can't say I blame them. I take a side-long look at myself as I pass The Gap. Despite the chill in the air, its plate-glass windows display bright summer fashions. And there, mirrored in the glass, among all the khaki splendor and colorful polo shirts, is my reflection. Clear as day. I caan waalk like a penguin! I turn beet red. I have adopted the penguin walk. Palms flat at the waist, wobbling back and forth, just like the goofy little girl in that old New England Aquarium TV ad.

What is going on with me today? I pull myself up and straighten my legs out. Or so I think. But at the next window I pass, I see the same stooped shuffle. The same penguin walk. There is no fooling myself. Whatever I did to myself last night in my sleep isn't going away. And scarily, I know that despite my jest, this situation is more serious than bad karma over mocking a commercial as a child.

At the next corner, I see the sign to my office building. I feel like I left my house three days ago and haven't eaten anything or drank fresh water since. I check my watch. It is 8:55. Just five minutes till work starts. I'm not ready to interact with the office crowd just yet, so, cursing the cobblestones, I shuffle to the north side of Faneuil Hall, where I find a deserted granite bench out of sight of my office and throw myself down. I pull my pack of cancer sticks out of my coat pocket, and torch another slim missile of death.

As I smoke the cigarette, I start to think of the strange numbness and have a light bulb moment. For about a month now, I have had problems with my shoes fitting correctly. I always feel my pinky toe on my left foot go numb and get trapped under my fourth toe. It has been bothering me so much that I recently bought bigger shoes. Now, I clomp around with shoes that are way too big and my pinky toe is still trapped. I wonder if that is related to this bizarre numbness.

I start to worry that this mysterious condition could take a turn for the worse, but what really bothers me is my math. This is only my fourth cigarette. I have not smoked the correct number of cigarettes by this point in the day. Believe it or not, I instinctually know I am behind schedule in the nicotine-fix column. What with the bizarre sensation in my legs and genitals, the long trip into work, and everything else, there is no way I can stray from my usual nicotine dosage this morning. If I am going to have any chance of being perceived as normal today, I have to consume that fifth cigarette.

Although it is my dream job, today, work can wait. I work for an up and coming residential real estate development firm. I am only the eighth person they hired, so the company is small and I wear a lot of hats. I'm also the youngest and have an opportunity that the Harvard kids would kill for. In the short six months that I have been with the company, I have really hit it off personally and professionally with everyone from the receptionist to the President and CEO. I plan on staying with this company for the long haul. This is my shot to make it and I don't want to risk that by taking frivolous days off.

I stand up, unsteady but I right myself as I pull out my pack, then sit back down and spark the crucial fifth cigarette. There aren't too many people walking around Faneuil Hall, mostly seniors and nannies off on their usual morning walk before the mass of consumers and tourists arrive at the old marketplace. All the business-types have disappeared into their lonely cubicles. After smoking two thirds of the cigarette, I have my fill and flick it in a sewer grate. I open my briefcase, grab my trusty bottle of cologne, and spray the fingers on my left hand to disguise the smoky smell. I pull out a stick of gum, pop it into my mouth, and make my way to the office.

Chapter Three - Just Another Day at the Office

As I exit the elevator, I see the company's sign on the glass wall entry way, right in front of me. The office is located in one of the oldest buildings in Faneuil Hall. The exposed brick walls and the sand blasted wood timbers in the ceiling are two hundred years old.

I check my feet one last time before my grand entrance. Everything looks normal. I don't want to let on to my bizarre condition. People will be busy, so I can sneak by unnoticed. I take a deep breath and pull the heavy glass door open. Still copying the penguin, I waddle in, using the wall as a guide. Right past the couch, the office takes a left, and then there is a gorgeous conference room with a full-length glass wall and a mahogany conference table.

The receptionist's desk, which is adjacent to the conference room, has a huge window behind it overlooking the popular Hong Kong bar. Sarah, the receptionist, sits behind her desk, already buried in her work. Her auburn ponytail is the only thing visible above the tall desk.

"Hey, Sarah," I say, slightly out of breath.

"Hey," she says, finishing her writing before glancing up at me. Then she drops her head back down to her work. I concentrate, step by step, leaving my finger prints on the glass conference room wall as I pass it.

Sarah glances up again. My progress is taking forever. The foyer seems longer than it ever has before. She looks up at me for a third time.

"You all right?" she asks loudly. She isn't exactly a delicate flower.

"Yeah, I'm fine," I mumble as I concentrated on my steps. I can hear someone stirring on the office side of the wall.

Gene pokes his head around the corner to see what was going on. "Mr. Matt!" he greets me. "You okay?"

"I'm fine," I say. "I slept wrong. Just a stiff back and neck, is all."

Gene is in his early fifties and has an athletic build. His graying hair is always pressed down and hat headed. He's our accountant/singer/songwriter/scratch golfer/Zen master. Although I haven't been on the job long, we share common interests and are forming a budding friendship. Plus, he has taken me under his wing and is showing me the ropes of real estate.

He studies me more closely. "Mr. Matt," he says, "you got a little limp working there."

"Yeah, it's bizarre. It's been like this all morning. I think maybe I did something to myself in my sleep last night and tweaked my back."

"Ouch! I've been there. So you don't think it's serious then?"

"Nah. I've had worse. This is more annoying than anything else. Why? What's up?"

"Well, I wanted to tell you that there is an opening in our group for this golf tournament on Friday. Gerard wants you to come."

My spirits instantly lift. Gerard is the owner of the company. In the six months I've been here, I didn't think he'd noticed me. This is my opportunity to schmooze with the owner. There is no way I can pass this opportunity up.

"Really? Wow. So Gerard wants me to play, huh?"

"Yeah, but, Matt, I don't know. You don't look so good." Gene helps me navigate around the moving boxes, cubicles, and filing cabinets toward my desk. In addition to Gene and Sarah, there are only three other people in the office. All pretending not to notice that I am walking like a penguin.

"If Gerard wants me there, I'll be there," I say with perhaps too much enthusiasm. "Besides, how long can

something like this possibly last? I'll be fine by Friday."
Friday is a long way away. Everything has to be fine.

~~~

I am a really regular, routine person. And by regular, I
mean regular. Okay … so I poop a lot. And right on
schedule, my stomach is now bubbling in an unsavory sea of
gas. The bathroom is placing a call that I have to answer. Or
else.

Fortunately, the level of cramping I am experiencing
gives me temporary superhuman strength, and I am able to
pull myself up and walk to the bathroom with barely any hint
of the penguin walk, or so I think.

Once inside the public bathroom, my good fortune
continues. There is no one else in the two-stall room. I dive
into the farthest stall, unbelt, detrouse, and sit down on the
seat. To my surprise everything flows fluidly. I am even able
to pee without straining. My momentary relief subsides,
however, when I realize I cannot feel anything coming out
from either side. The proof is below me in the toilet, but the
usual sensations that accompany a strenuous movement are
absent.

Now I am really starting to feel anxious on top of my
confusion. Normal things like going to the bathroom and
walking are not so normal anymore. The part that is
bothering me the most is that my condition is visibly
noticeable. I'm not the type of person who likes to be noticed.
I like to go about my business behind the scenes and let my
actions do the talking.

I certainly don't want to miss anytime from work while
I am trying to get established with this company. I am not
going to blow it over a case of numbness. I have worked
damn hard to earn my ticket to this white-collar life. And I
am going to work even harder now that I have this

opportunity.

This is why I don't call-in or go home sick even on days like this. However, this condition is not getting any better. For the first time today, I realize that something must be seriously wrong with me. I know that I am going to have to ask for help. It is time to talk to the boss. I get up off the toilet, wash my hands and struggle to do the impossible.

Bob is in his fifties, reserved and very intuitive. He is the strong, silent type who doesn't say much, but when he does, you listen. I am extremely intimidated by him but know that he is best person in the office to go to for an issue this serious.

"Hey, Bob, can we go talk?"

He looks over at me. Even though he is giving me a blank stare, I know he is picking up a lot. God only knows what kind of vibes I am throwing off right now. I shouldn't have said anything.

"Yeah, sure," he says, without smiling. "Is there anyone in the conference room?"

I don't know for sure, but I take a guess. "I think it's free."

"Okay," he says turning back to his computer monitor. "Give me a minute, and I'll meet you over there."

I pull myself up and slowly make my way into the conference room. Not only is Bob my boss, but he is also the CEO of the company. My mind starts racing. Should I even be bringing him in on this personal matter? Where do you start with something like this? *Bob, I can't feel my feet, legs, and penis.* My heart starts beating too fast again. I can feel myself getting even more anxious and flushed.

Bob arrives moments later and wastes no time. "What's up?" he asks.

"Well...I don't know how to put this, Bob, but I've got no feeling in my legs."

Bob looks at me puzzled.

I try to explain. "You know, um, well, it's kind of funny. You know … when you sit on something wrong for a long time, you get that pins and needles feeling?"

"Un huh." He nods.

"Well, it's like that, only it won't go away."

Bob hesitates before trying to gather more details. "This is your legs you're talking about? I thought you said earlier that it was just a stiff back?"

From the look in his eyes, I can tell that I have his full attention. He leans in toward me and pulls his lip, focusing intently on my every word. One thing I have learned about working with guys in their fifties is that they can be very open about their health. Sensing compassion, I share more embarrassing details of my morning struggle.

"It started when I woke up this morning. I was completely numb from the waist down. I keep thinking it will get better, but it hasn't stopped. I mean, it hasn't gotten any better. The feeling's just not going away, I mean, I don't have any feeling, you know, the feeling that I have no feeling…."

Bob looks puzzled as I ramble on.

"It's been, like, a couple of hours now, and it's just not going away." I am now repeating myself like a complete idiot.

"Really, Matt," Bob's face now registers great concern. "You have to go to the doctor to get this checked out."

After spilling my guts, I am breathing easier. The edge is off my anxiety. Of course, that's always when I slip back into the macho Italian mode.

"Yeah," I answer in my strongest voice, "I don't want to get too overly dramatic here. I can finish the day."

Bob sits up straight in his chair like a judge ready to deliver a verdict. "Here's what you do," he says in a clear, commanding voice. "You call your doctor's office right now and tell them what's going on. They'll let you know what you have to do next."

He leans on the table and looks at me. "If I were you, I'd go see your doctor now. This could be a circulatory issue. Or something more serious. You need to be evaluated. You don't mess around with something like this."

Knowing he is right, I pull my cell phone out of my pocket, along with my insurance ID card. I dial the number on the card and am connected to my primary healthcare office. Confident that I am doing the right thing, Bob nods and leaves the room. After the usual back and forth banter with my ID number, I am finally connected to a nurse and describe my symptoms. Well, most of my symptoms that is. My awkward sleeping penis syndrome and the lack of feeling when using the bathroom are way too embarrassing for me to share with a strange woman over the phone.

"You say it's like a pins and needles sensation?" she asks.

"Yeah. I can't feel anything."

"But you decided you would go into work and not to the doctor this morning?"

She has me on that one. "Umm, yeah."

"I see," she says quietly.

"Well, what do you think it is?"

"Tell me, did you do any heavy lifting recently? Yard work? Weight lifting? You know, things of that nature."

"Yeah we're moving from one office to another at work and I go to gym every other day," I reply.

"Well, honey, given your symptoms, it sounds like you have pinched a nerve in your back. Unfortunately, the best remedy is Tylenol and time."

"Really?" I look down at my legs. "That's it, huh? Tylenol and rest? Who knew?"

"Well, if it does persist for more than the next forty-eight hours or so, come on in and see us."

I breathe a sigh of relief. "Thank you so much for your help."

"If I were you," she said, "I would tell your boss and call it a day. Go home and put your feet up. That may help."

"Thanks. Thanks again."

"You take care now," she says, and hangs up the phone.

Wow. Is that all this is? What a relief. Man, I was going through all of this for a pinched nerve? I didn't tell her about the penis thing, but that probably comes with the pinched nerve, too. I've never had a pinched nerve. That is probably it. Pins and needles in the feet. The legs. And a limp penis. Okay, I don't want to think about that one too much. I make my way back to my desk and relay my findings to Bob. He smiles at my relief. I tell him that I'll stick it out for the rest of the day because there is nothing I can do but let it heal. Who knew? There really is a magical pill and it goes by the name of Tylenol. Sign me up!

Chapter Four - Numbing End to Numbing Day

The return commute home is every bit as grueling as the morning. To add insult to injury, I add nearly an hour to my route by back tracking from North Quincy into Dorchester to catch the highway because it is the flattest possible route home. My willingness to take risks has dramatically decreased by this point in the day.

With tremendous relief, I pull into the driveway of our home just before seven o'clock. The house is dark. Jocelyn's Mustang isn't there. She must still be at the gym. I fire up one last smoke and sit in my truck. That's when I remember that I forgot to call Jocelyn to tell her I am not going to the gym.

I sigh and take another puff. Usually, I do the cooking but there is no way that I can tonight. Tonight I'm not even hungry. I just need some sleep. And some more Tylenol. Extra-strength, please.

I take a last deep inhale of the smoke and flick the butt out the window, watching the cherry ember flicker on the way to the ground. The last drag is always my favorite. As I'm smoking a cigarette, my mind just skips along and I tell myself, I'm gonna quit, I'm gonna quit, I'm gonna quit. But when the last drag comes with its final fireworks flicker, I tell myself, "One more won't kill me."

Climbing ever so slowly out of the cab, I waddle away from my truck and haltingly climb the five steps to the front door. The door creaks as I enter the house. I drop my briefcase at the door and penguin-walk to the kitchen.

No need for lights. Jocelyn keeps a clean, orderly house. There are no hidden obstacles along the way. As I walk through the dining room, the headlights from commuters heading home shine through the picture window, painting my path down the hallway. I arrive in our bedroom and collapse on the bed, mentally and physically exhausted.

~~~

"Matty?"

I feel someone shaking my shoulder.

"What's wrong?" Jocelyn's voice has an air of concern. Warm drool wets my cheek. My face is buried in our fluffy down comforter.

I look up. "Wrong? Uh ... nothing's wrong ... why?" I'm still groggy. "I must have fallen asleep."

I roll over to face her. The room is completely dark. All I can see is her silhouette. She sits beside me on the bed.

"Matt, you left the front door wide open and you're lying on the bed with your shoes on. What's going on?"

"Yeah," I mumble, stroking her leg. "About the shoes. I think I need your help getting them off."

"Why? What's wrong?" She runs her fingers through my hair. I feel like I'm talking to her in a dream.

"How can I explain this? Umm. I woke up this morning and my feet were asleep. Then when I was in the shower, I realized that it was more than my feet. It was everything below my waist. I mean, everything."

A startled look comes over her face. "Matt, you aren't making any sense. What do you mean everything's asleep? You didn't say anything this morning?"

I reach out and grab her hand. "I know. I know. I didn't want to worry you. I thought it would just go away. But it didn't. I called my doctor's office, and the nurse I spoke to said it was probably a pinched nerve in my back and to just take some Tylenol. It should be better tomorrow."

Jocelyn's shoulders relax as she exhales. She strokes the back of my hand. "A pinched nerve, huh. I told you that you probably overdid it at the gym. You need to be careful. You always try to do too much. I'll make you dinner tonight.

What do you feel like?"

I groan. "I'm not really hungry. I just want to take some Tylenol PM. I think all I need is a good night's sleep. Hopefully, I'm better tomorrow morning."

She laughs. "You're not hungry? There must be something really wrong with you!"

I push her away playfully, and go back to hugging my pillow. She gets up to get me the Tylenol PM and some water. In what feels like only a second, she's back with a glass of water and some pills in her hand.

I sit up and take everything like a good boy. The recommended dosage is two tablets, but since I'm a big guy in pain, Jocelyn thinks three will do the trick. She then takes off my shoes and helps me undress. She's so patient. She'll make a wonderful mother some day. She grabs the remote and turns on an *Everybody Loves Raymond* rerun for me. I lean back against my pillow. As everybody in the Romano family complains and yells to the laugh track, I slowly drift off into a medically-induced sleep, hoping that by tomorrow everything will be back to normal.

Chapter Five - Thursday, May 19

It is about a quarter till seven in the morning. I'm lying half awake, half in a fog, out on the living room couch, looking up out the window at my neighbor's pesky pine with its enormous low-hanging branches blowing dangerously towards my direction. I am definitely grumpy this morning, increasing my hatred for that friggin' tree. Since the day we moved in here, I've worried that a good storm will topple it over and destroy our house and vehicles. Plus, it's a bitch to pick up all the pinecones and needles it sprinkles in our yard. But there's nothing I can do about it. It's in my neighbor's yard, and she is a sweet elderly woman who lives alone. So I tolerate her damn tree.

I tossed and turned most of the night in bed. Despite our cozy pillow top queen bed, I couldn't get comfortable. At some point in the middle of the night, I retreated to the couch to sleep with my legs elevated on the foot rest. My hope was that sleeping on my back and elevating my legs, along with some more extra-strength Tylenol, would help alleviate the pinched nerve symptoms thus restoring my legs to their rightful pre-pins-and-needles condition.

I was dead wrong.

My condition did not improve. In fact, I seem to be more lethargic than ever. I must have really overdone it yesterday. I know I should probably take it easy today and not go into work but I don't want to jeopardize my spot in the golf tournament tomorrow. I probably need to give the Tylenol at least twenty-four hours to kick in. I guess expecting my condition to completely go away overnight was a little too optimistic. Now time to motivate myself for another exhausting commute. I flip the TV channel to the news, hoping for at least some sunshine to get me through this day.

No such luck. Intermittent showers and thick cloud cover. Perfect. Another sloppy commute. My morning weather reports were sure different in Arizona. Actually, in Arizona, I didn't need to watch weather reports at all because it was always sunny. So why'd we move back here again? Oh, yeah. The three F's: friends, family and the four seasons. Turns out they are all overrated.

Jocelyn is standing over me now, already dressed for work, her blown-dry hair bouncing off her shoulders. Her eyes are filled with concern.

"Come here." I murmur. "I was just day dreaming about us in warm, sunny Arizona."

I twist sideways so my back is against the back of the couch and open the blanket, inviting her to join me. She smiles and crawls under the blanket, with her face to mine, and kisses me gently on the lips.

"I don't want to think about the weather, baby. It's way too depressing. So why'd you sleep out here last night?" she asks, changing the subject.

"I just couldn't get comfortable. So I came out here to watch TV."

"Poor baby. The Tylenol didn't do anything?"

"No, not yet."

"Really? Are your legs any better today at all?" She tries to be optimistic, but can tell by the look in my eyes. Nothing's improved.

I shake my head. "It's the strangest thing I think I've ever gone through. I mean ... it's not any worse, but it's not any better at all. To tell you the truth, I'm starting to get a little scared."

She puts her hand on my cheek. "Don't you think this is probably a good time to go see the doctor? I know the nurse said it's a pinch nerve but what if she's wrong. They can't diagnose you over the phone."

"I just started taking the Tylenol yesterday." I say, shifting my weight. "I'm going to try and go to work again. There's a golf tournament tomorrow for work. Gerard invited me to it. I don't want to go to the doctor's and have him tell me that I can't golf."

She gives me a hard but compassionate look. "I am not a doctor and I can tell you that you shouldn't be golfing. Pinched nerve or whatever- golfing is a bad idea."

I chuckle, but I can tell she's getting more than a little frustrated with me. "Baby," I tell her, "you don't call in sick to a golf tourney. Ever! Especially if playing means I'll have a chance to impress the owner of the company."

She gives me a very skeptical stare. She's not afraid to call me out on my bullshit excuses. "And you expect me to believe that drinking beers and playing golf with a bad back is somehow going to help your future with this company?"

Yeah, she has a point. And I have one, too. Although I'm losing sight of what it is. I seem to be losing a lot of things lately.

Chapter Six - Boss Knows Best

After another grueling ride to work, Bob and I are in the conference room again. Before I have a chance to put my briefcase down, he wants an update on my situation. He must think that I am crazy to attempt work two days in a row with this strange condition. I am starting think that I am crazy, too. His eyes are like a white hot spotlight on me. Even though I know this is health-related, I still feel like a kid being called into the principal's office.

Bob starts. "So, is it any better?" His poker face belies his concern.

"Things are pretty much the same but that commute completely wiped me out. I didn't think I was going to make it. It is taking more and more strength just to take one simple step." I pause and look down at my legs. Then I look up and into his eyes. "Not only can I not feel my legs, but I'm having trouble going to the bathroom."

"What do you mean? Are you constipated?" He is looking at me very intently.

I almost start to laugh because I'm not sure I've ever had this conversation with another human being. Especially my boss. I compose myself. This is serious.

Okay, breathe.

"It's not really constipation," I finally say. "It's different than that." Feeling that I can trust him, I decide to push all of my chips into the pot. "The thing is, Bob ... I can't feel anything down there."

"Really? You can't feel anything?"

I shake and lower my head in embarrassment and disbelief.

Bob is speechless, pulling on his lower lip. I can tell that he is searching for the right thing to say.

"Matt," he finally utters in a compassionate but stern voice. "If you're having trouble in the bathroom, this is very, very serious. You need to go talk to someone right away. This sounds like more than a pinched nerve to me."

He pauses looking alarmed. "I want you to go to the doctor today. Don't worry about work. Everything here can wait. With the condition you're in, you probably shouldn't golf tomorrow, either"

"Bob," I start my rebuttal

"Matt," his voice is firm as he cuts me off, "you need to go to the doctor now."

The way he looks, I know he means business.

"Okay," I sigh.

He pats me on the back as he stands up to leave the room. "Now would be a good time."

I am not excited about leaving work and going to the doctor, but that's what Bob wants me to do. I don't want to rock the boat, so I penguin-walk back to my desk and pack up my stuff.

Gene is standing over my desk. "Hey, Matt," he says, "I've gotta run out to the bank. Where are you off to?"

"Bob thinks I need to see the doctor. I think I'm fine. But whatever...."

"I think Bob might be on to something there. Here let me help you." Gene throws my bag over his shoulder and helps me past the line of sympathetic onlookers.

In a small office, the rumor mill of my condition is running rampant. Everyone wants to know how I am doing. My answer to all is the same. "You know how when you fall asleep on your arm and you get those pins and needles feelings? Well, that's what my legs are like."

It's hard to describe to people what you are going through when on the outside you don't look sick. I don't want to be different. Not now. So far, I fit in at this company and I don't want anything to jeopardize that.

Chapter Seven - Urgent Care

As I take a seat in the waiting room of the Medical Center's Urgent Care Clinic, I feel all of my weight drip into the chair. I hadn't realized how tired I am until now. My feet might as well be made of wood. At this point, I am moving my feet and legs completely by memory of how they are supposed to move. If I don't get my feeling back soon, I am going to be in big trouble. How much longer can this muscle memory last?

I close my eyes for a few moments, open them again and pick up the newspaper on the waiting room table next to me. I immediately flip to the classifieds and scan the ads about puppies for sale.

"Matthew Cavallo."

That was quick. I put the paper down on the seat next to me, stand up, and penguin-walk down the hall behind the nurse. She is walking five feet in front of me at a hurried pace, so she doesn't see me using the walls to support myself. She leads me into an exam room, closes the door behind her, and tells me to sit on the exam table. Thus begins the standard examination routine.

"What brings you in today, Matthew? Open wide. I'm going to take your temperature."

I sit on the table and the paper crinkles under me as I shift my weight. I open my mouth as wide as possible and stare around the room. It is your typical bland examining room with cheap paintings and framed diplomas.

When she takes the thermometer from my mouth, I answer her first question. "I think it's a pinched nerve. Everything from the waist down is asleep. When I say everything, I mean everything."

"That's unusual," she replies. "Did you do anything to

your back that you remember? I'm going to take your blood pressure now. Roll up your left sleeve."

I do as I am told. "I can't remember specifically doing anything," I say. "But I do go to the gym, and I was working on my yard this past weekend. Plus, I was moving some heavy stuff at work. So that might be it."

"Your blood pressure is high."

"I smoke and I had a couple coffees today," I answer. "That probably doesn't help."

"No, it doesn't," she says, pursing her lips. She jots notes on my chart and walks to the door, stopping with her hand on the knob. "I'll let the doctor know you're here," she says, and then she is gone.

That's it? What did she write on my chart, I barely said anything? Was it wrong to say I smoke? Everybody knows that smoking is a terrible habit. Even I know that. Now that I've spilled my guts, the insurance companies will have that information in their greedy little hands.

There is a knock on the door and, after I shout out a greeting, the good doctor walks in. Dr. Chalko is a quirky little man. Small in stature, bald on top, with some dark hair clinging for life to the sides of his head. As he crosses the room, I realize that he is not looking directly at me, but rather looking toward me in an anxious way. Even so, I try to be friendly, as is my nature.

"Hi, Dr. Chalko."

"Matt." He moves into position in front of me. "What is the problem today?" He looks down at my chart. "The nurse says you are experiencing some numbness in your legs?"

"It's the weirdest thing, Dr. Chalko. You know that pins and needles feeling you get when you sit on something for too long? Well, it's like that. My foot's asleep. Both feet. As well as my legs and…" I blush "…I think my genitals, too."

There is a moment of silence. He looks at the clipboard

as if something is written on it in a foreign language that he can't read.

"Your genitals? What do you mean exactly?"

"Well, I'm having trouble urinating. I find that I really have to strain in order to make myself go. If I eventually can go, I can see it come out, but I can't feel it."

His face remains buried in the clipboard. "Is it only your penis?" he asks.

"Yeah." Then I remember. "Wait. No. I had a bowel movement yesterday, but I didn't feel anything in that area, either." This is just about the most humiliating disclosure of my life. My face must be beet red.

"Okay," he says, still giving me nothing. He reaches into his jacket. "I'm going to test your reflexes now."

He pulls a little mallet out of his pocket, bends over my right knee like he is expecting a cuckoo bird to pop out, and strikes it right in the middle. I don't feel anything, but the damned knee still responds and kicks out a bit. He then does the same thing to my left knee, with the same results. He then goes on to do the other reflex tests. My body keeps responding normally. Well, at least according to my definition of normal. It's not really normal when your reflexes respond, but you can't feel the rubber hammer.

Dr. Chalko seems uneasy. "I've got to make a phone call," he says, and with that, he is out the door, looking down at his clipboard as he exits.

A phone call? I still have no idea what is going on and he is making a phone call! I need something to quiet my racing mind so I reach over to the metal chair next to the exam table and pick up an out-of-date golf magazine. What could be more boring than reading about golf? Just as I am scanning the contents page, Dr. Chalko comes back into the room without knocking.

"Sorry about that," he says, slightly disheveled looking.

"No problem. Am I gonna make it, Doc?" I say with a

laugh.

He completely ignores my attempt at humor. "What I'm going to need you to do is take down your pants and roll over and face the wall."

Whoa … this guy really doesn't have a sense of humor. Or maybe it is a lot more warped than I think. I give him a puzzled look, but he is completely serious, so I do as I am told. The paper crinkles again as I awkwardly pull my pants down while seated on the table. Then I turn over and faced the wall.

"I need you to pull down your underwear," he says.

I struggle with my boxers, pulling them down over my thighs. It is difficult enough with my numb legs, not to mention lying sideways on an exam table with that crinkly paper. By this time, I figure out that I am going to be receiving my first rectal examination. Twenty-eight years old, and my very first time. I've heard all the jokes about it, but I never really thought the day would come. Well, here it is. I am almost glad I wasn't given a heads-up. Almost.

I hear the latex glove snap on his hand. He coughs as if he is embarrassed as he prepares to examine me. There is a faint smell of rubber. Then, without hesitation, he steals my anal virginity. I stare desperately at the walls for something to take my mind off this awkward encounter but all I see is the blank screen of white painted walls illuminated by soft lighting. Nothing to take my mind off his probing fingers.

Then it hits me. I can't feel his finger. I mean, in me. Why can't I feel his finger in me! He is up against me, his coat almost hanging in my face. In fact, I can feel his hot breath. He is exerting himself as he probes. But I can't feel him in me! Here I am with one, possibly two, fingers up my ass, and I can't feel a damn thing. I am so confused- I don't WANT to feel a guy's finger up my ass but I SHOULD be feeling this!

The sound of the doctor snapping the glove off impedes my emotional meltdown. For now, anyway. He steps on the trash can lever, and when the lid pops up, throws it in. "I have to make another phone call."

I fumble as I turn myself around to face him, while simultaneously trying to pull my pants back up. "Doctor, can you give me some idea what's going on?"

"I am going to call a neurologist and try to get you scheduled as soon as possible," he says as he moves to the door. "You can get dressed now." And then he is gone again.

I wiggle enough on the table to finish pulling my pants back up and buckle my belt. I lie and wonder why I just didn't jump off the table and get dressed normally. There is just such an unreal atmosphere to this examination room. It is a little bit like *Alice Through the Looking Glass*.

To my surprise, the doctor comes back into the room as quickly as he left it. This time he looks at me. "Matt, I just spoke with Dr. Kumar at Neurology Associates. He wants you to call and schedule an appointment as soon as you leave here. It is important that he see you at his first possible opening."

What? My head is spinning. I say the first thing that pops into my head. "Dr. Chalko, I smoke. Do you think this could be a circulatory issue?"

He hesitates, as if he is deciding whether or not he should talk to me at all. "No," he says slowly. "I think you may have a condition called Transverse Myelitis." He holds up his hands, as if he senses I am about to bombard him with a ton of questions. "This is just a guess. But your symptoms seem to be in line with that condition."

Needless to say, I am more than a little stunned and more confused than ever.

"What is this trans—whatever thing you said?"

He smiles but this is not another one of my attempts at humor. I really can't remember what he said. "Transverse Myelitis," he repeats. "Dr. Kumar will tell you about it."

"Okay," I mumble, too overwhelmed to press any further.

"He'll be expecting your call. Make sure you call right away."

"Okay, Dr Chalko. Thanks."

He extends his hand, giving me a piece of paper. This is Dr. Kumar's number," he says.

I nod and take the slip of paper.

He pulls his hand back and looks down. "Good luck, Matthew." And then he is gone. This time for good.

Clutching the neurologist's phone number, I feel like I am in a fog. What do I do now? I am physically and mentally drained and not any closer to getting my legs fixed. I didn't even write down what the doctor said. What is it again, trans something or other? Think, Matt, think! I can't remember for the life of me. By the time I get to the Medical Center's front door, the trans whatever is just a sound in my head and has lost all meaning. I really think I blew it now. I go see the doctor and I can't remember what he said so now I have to worry about what it might be. Can trans what-you-may-call-it be another name for a pinched nerve? It sounds serious and I'm pissed at myself for not being more assertive and for not making Dr. Chalko explain it to me. I'm hopeless.

I climb into my truck and pull out the crumbled piece of paper from my pocket.

Dr. Kumar.

This is going to be interesting.

I dial my cell phone.

"Good afternoon, Neurology Associates."

Deep breath. "Hi, I need to make an appointment with Dr. Kumar."

"Have you been in to see him before?"

"No. I just left the Medical Center. I was referred to you guys by Dr. Chalko."

Rustling paper.

"Let me see."

More rustling paper.

"We have an opening on June 21st. Will that work for you?"

"June 21st? That's almost a month away. Dr. Chalko just told me he talked to Dr. Kumar and that I need to be seen as soon as possible. I can't wait that long! I can't feel my legs." I am not going to be so passive now, not after I screwed up with Dr. Chalko.

Pause on the other end.

"I see. What is your name?"

"Matthew Cavallo. C A V, as in Victor, A L L O."

"Okay, hold on one moment."

I hold. I take her words as not just a momentary pause in our phone conversation, but also as advice. I try to catch my breath as the smooth sounds of Magic 106.7 sings in my ear. But Luther Vandross isn't doing it for me today.

The music stops.

"Matthew, sorry about the wait. Is Monday at 4:20 good for you?"

I sigh with relief. "Yeah, that sounds good. Thanks. I appreciate it. I'll see you then."

I hang up the phone and rest my head against the steering wheel.

Why do I need a brain doctor? The feet are about as far away from the brain as you can get. I grab a pen out of the glove box and scribble the appointment on a scrap of paper I find on the passenger seat. I've already forgotten the diagnosis. I am not taking any chances on forgetting the doctor who is going to fix me.

Dr. Kumar at 4:20 P.M.

I pause.

"Funny.." I chuckle. *Harold and Kumar go to White Castle.*"

That is one of my and Jocelyn's favorite movies. The movie's main character, Kumar, is headed for medical school, but he puts it off to smoke pot and get into compromising comical situations with his best friend, Harold. Seeing as the police code, and now universal slang, for pot is 420, the irony of meeting Dr. Kumar at 4:20 is beyond coincidence. I guess God does have a sense of humor after all.

Chapter Eight - Friday, May 20

It is a cold, cloudy, wet, and windy day. Not ideal conditions for golfing. The only positive is that the weather gives me another excuse for how poorly I am about to play. I am feeling a little guilty for being out on the golf course today. Not only has there been no improvement in my condition, but I also just lied to my wife. Before Jocelyn left for work, I assured her that there was no way I was going to play golf today. Not only that, but that I wouldn't drive or leave the house. Then as soon as she left the house, I got ready and left. Call it what you will, but you don't call in sick to a golf tournament. Ever.

As I limp up to the clubhouse, I see golf carts lined up two by two along the side of the building and people spilling out of the community room, grabbing their clubs, and heading toward the carts. I take a breather and set the golf bag in the rack and lean against the fence. Everyone else seems to be getting ready for the start.

"Hey, Matt, you need a beer for the course?" a voice yells from the clubhouse door.

"Sure. Grab me a Sam's Summer," I say in my best macho voice. I start up again, grabbing my golf bag and slinging it over my shoulder. But this time the weight of it nearly knocks me over. My knees buckle. I reach for the bag rack to steady myself.

What the hell am I getting myself into? Once I regain my balance, I head toward the course, walking like a penguin again. Most of the tournament participants are standing alongside their assigned carts. Wafts of cigar smoke float in the air. Golf clubs clack as they are inspected on the backs of the carts.

I head down the aisle of golf carts, trying to make it to

my cart without being noticed. Then I see Bob two carts over, motioning to me. "You're playing with me, Gene, and Walter," he says.

Damn. No Gerard. I thought this morning would be my moment to bond with the owner of the company, my one chance for him to get to know me better. Oh well, I've come too far to turn back now and it is still a bonding opportunity with my boss.

I secure the clubs on the back of the cart and climb into the passenger side, trying to ignore the numbness of my legs and feet. Walter makes his way toward me and hands me a frosty cold beer in a plastic cup.

"Thanks, Walter. This is exactly what I need." I take a big chug and wipe the foam off my lip. Walter sits down in Bob's cart, so that must mean I am with Gene. At least I will have the pleasure of watching probably the best player in the field at today's tournament.

"Hey, Matt, how are the legs today?" Gene asks as he slides into the driver's seat of our cart.

"Hey," I reply. "Um ... the same."

"So, really, no improvement huh? Should you even be playing golf? If it were me in your shoes, I wouldn't have left the house."

Funny, it seems I am hearing that a lot lately. Not only that, but I can feel Bob eyeing me from the next cart.

"Matt. The doctor. What did he say?" Bob joins in with obvious interest.

Oh shit. He remembers my appointment. I look around and see all eyes focused on me. I am put on-the-spot and I have to say something. Usually, in these spots I go for a joke, but gauging the concern on the face of my coworkers, I decide to come straight with it.

"Well, they want me to see a neurologist. I'm not even sure what a neurologist does. Or why I would have to see a brain doctor for numbness in my lower half?" I shrug.

Bob looks me straight in the eye. "Really, a neurologist? This sounds like it is more serious than a pinched nerve. I'm really not sure that you should be out here golfing today."

I met his eyes. "Bob, I can do this. I promise the second something doesn't feel right, I'll go home." But something already doesn't feel right- the numbness.

He pauses for a second. A long second. Then he leans back in his cart. "Okay. Whatever you've got to do, we'll understand."

The tournament is a standard scramble. I listen from my seat in Gene's cart as the tournament director spells out the rules. We all drive from the tee box, the best drive is selected, and then we play the best shot into the cup.

"We're starting on the seventh hole today," Gene says, looking at the instruction sheet clipped to his steering wheel.

The tournament is a shotgun start, meaning that all players start at the same time, only at different holes. All of a sudden, the carts ahead of us jump forward, and Gene pushes our cart out onto the path, in search of the seventh hole. The morning mist is cold against my face as we wind through the course, following the trail of golf carts. Gene is good at reading people and knows that I want to avoid talking about my legs at all cost so he keeps the conversation light with talk of sports and weather.

We pull up to our tee box. It is a 121-yard par three with a sand trap protecting the front of the green, with trees behind to the right. All in all, it is a pretty safe shot to the green if you carry the trap, but there are thick cranberry bogs beyond the green to the left.

"Go ahead, Matt," Gene says. "Why don't you get us started. A soft nine iron is all you need."

Yeah, easy for him to say, he could be playing on the tour. I grab a hold of the roof bar of the cart and pull myself out. The cart lurches considerably, but I try to ignore it. Then

I hold onto the side of the cart as I penguin-walk to the back.

I grab the eight iron to be safe and waddle over to the tee box. Using the club as a crutch, I bend down on one knee and insert a tee into the ground. I am about to lose my balance and spin to the earth in a heap, but I miraculously right myself and even manage to place the ball on the tee. Then I push myself up and address the ball. I don't know how many swings I have in me, so I am not going to waste a good one on a practice swing. The guys stand behind me and watch. I stand with my feet shoulder-length apart and bend my knees slightly.

I can't get comfortable. I grip my hands tightly around the club, extend the club from my body and raise it slowly back. Then I drop my shoulder and swing, but as I do, my hips lock. I look up just in time to see my ball pop straight up in the air and plop into the red abyss of the cranberry bog just to the left of us.

"That was weird," I say, as I step away from the tee box, "I couldn't get my hips to turn. I'm completely locked up."

"That's ok, Matt," Gene says, "It's best ball, so we'll use another team member's shot. Just get into the cart and rest."

"I'm fine guys, really. My hips just locked."

Unfortunately, swing after swing, it is the same result. I want to swing, but my legs will not turn and pivot. As a result, I have to swing the club with just my upper body, and any golfer will tell you, that spells disaster. As the day wears on, my new legless swing is draining my energy and patience, and I find myself sitting in the cart more and more. The guys are being super supportive, but at this moment, I know something is seriously wrong with me.

After more than four hours of humiliating folly, we stand in the tee box of our last hole, the sixth. Under the scramble rules, we have to use at least one drive from each player. I have swung so badly on the last seventeen holes that we are down to the last one and still haven't used any of my drives. Gene is on the tee box, surveying the hole. He turns to me.

"Mr. Matt," he says, "just take a nice smooth seven iron and lay one out there. Then I can go over the trees and go for it." He points at the tree line.

The sixth hole is a 275-yard par four that doglegs right before the green. The green is protected by trees, but the fairway is open and hazard free, with the exception of a sand trap just before a cranberry bog at the far left of the fairway. Anyone who has seen my round thus far today knows that I have already squashed enough cranberries to put Ocean Spray out of business.

I take a deep breath and address the ball. The guys need my drive. I have to deliver. Concentrating on the ball, I bring my club back, drop my shoulder, and swing through the ball. It sounds good off the club.

"It's leaking a little left," Walter yells. "Stay in play, you son of a bitch!"

I pull my head up but I can't see the ball. "Where is it?"

Walter points toward the bog.

"Oh shit." I feel like I just let the world down.

"You might be all right," Bob reassures me. "Let's go check it out."

There is no point in anyone else hitting their drives. To follow the rules, we have to use my drive. So we climb into our carts and lurch back onto the cart path.

I am so embarrassed. We need to use my drive and it is looking like I have lost another ball in the bogs. Damn! I can't bear it. We ride toward my ball in silence. Then I see it.

It isn't in the cranberry bog. It hit the trap and is semi-buried in the sand two feet from the ominous lip. Some golfers would call my ball a fried egg because of the way it is partially buried in the sand.

"Breakfast ball, eh?" Gene, says, riffing off the fried egg notion. "That'll do, Mr. Matt. We can play it."

"Great," I mumble. How in the hell am I going to take a hack at the ball? I mean, it is in the worst possible place for me. The side of a hill buried in sand.

Gene parks the golf cart on an angle of a small hill and jumps out. I pull myself out of the cart, using the roof bar, but without Gene sitting in the other side, the cart almost tips over on me. It is like getting out of a bucking boat on the high seas. I miscalculate the distance to the ground and stumble back, slamming my hip into the cart. This is the only time in the last few days that I am glad that I can't feel anything. I grab my seven iron, then turn to face the incline of grass to the trap. I start shuffling up the little hill, using the seven iron as a cane. In my imagination, I am seeing myself doing my best pimp-strut imitation as I approach the ball. But intellectually, I know there is nothing cool or suave about my movements right now.

After dropping their balls into the sand trap next to mine, the guys each take their shots.

Gene senses my predicament. "Mr. Matt, I'm safely on the green. Not as close as I'd like to be, but still ... I think we can go ahead and pick up your ball."

I wave him off. "Nope. I've been looking at this shot for a while. I think I have a bead on it," I say bravely.

I stop and look at Gene, then look at the ball. "I can get it there, Gene."

He pauses again, like he is checking himself from saying something. Then he smiles. "Ok, let's see it."

I drop my right foot into the sand with my left above the trap's lip on the grass. I try to twist my right foot to plant it firmly in the sand, but my right ankle rolls. And just like that, I find myself lying sideways in the sand. I go down like a sack of potatoes dropped from the back end of a flatbed truck. I hear the peanut gallery hold back their laughs. I twist my neck and look up at them.

"Go ahead. Say it. I told you so."

The laughter explodes. I close my eyes in embarrassment. Why couldn't I just stop when I had the chance? I flail around like a beached whale as I try to get up out of the sand. I attempt to joke my way out of it. "Is someone going to help me up? Or take a picture, at least?"

Gene steps into the trap, grabs my arm, and yanks me up. As I dust myself off, he leans down quickly and scoops my ball out of the sand. Without a word, I take it as quickly as he hands it to me and stuff it in my pocket.

Gene's ball is laying about twenty-five feet from the hole. We stand behind the putt. It is a tough, slightly uphill, twenty-five-footer that seems to break hard, left to right. Walter steps up. He pulls his putter back and hits the ball toward the hole. It is right on line.

"It's got a chance," I yell. "It's got a chance! Oh, Oh, Oh!"

The putt falls just a couple inches short. Walter walks up and marks the ball.

"Thanks for showing us the way," Bob says as he lines up his putt. He leans over the ball and strokes it but it leaks left of the hole and short.

"What do you think, Matt?" Gene says. "It's down to me and you."

"Let me go," I say. "You've been lights out today. You should go last to save us."

He nods. "A little advice, though" he says. "All you have to do is get in touch with it. Stop thinking. Let things happen. Be the ball."

I smile. That last one is from *Caddyshack*, just to loosen me up. *Be the ball, Matty.*

I have just watched Walter and Bob show me the way to the hole. The layout reveals itself to me. Standing behind the putt, I think I see a crease in the green that rolls from where the ball is to the hole. The only thing I need to do is give it some speed, and that crease will take it home. I look at the putt again. Yeah, that makes sense. *Be the ball.* I line up, bring the putter back, and swing through the ball like a precise pendulum. The ball travels flawlessly down the line, curving slightly with the break.

"Be it," I say quietly. The line is perfect, but it looks like it is coming in a little too hot. My heart pops into my throat. "Beeeeee IT."

Shit! It is right on line. Does it have too much steam? The ball hits the back of the hole and pops up in the air. Time stops. We hold our collective breath. Then it drops straight in the center of the cup.

"IT'S IN THE HOLE!" I give the Tiger Woods fist pump. Everyone pounds my back. This is what I have been waiting for all day. A flash of brilliance and to be one of the guys. Finally. This is a good twenty-five-footer. "Great shot, Matt," Gene says, patting me on the back. We all shake hands over the cup and return back toward the carts.

We drop off our clubs, park our carts, and head to the clubhouse for dinner. I am bone-tired from the long day, plus, I am wet and sandy from my escapade in the trap. Too tired to continue my worn-thin charade any longer.

I clear my throat. "Thanks for putting up with me today, guys," I mumble.

"What? Was something wrong?" Gene jokes. "I thought you always shot like that."

I smile at him. I am feeling great after that heroic putt, but I know I have to stop fooling myself. I have nothing left. I turn to Bob. "I don't think I'm going to stick around for the dinner," I tell him. "I feel kind of weak."

Bob looks relieved. "That's probably the smartest thing you've said all day."

Chapter Nine - Monday, May 23

"Matthew Cavallo," a doctor with an Indian accent calls out to the waiting room of the neurology office. I drop my outdated *Sports Illustrated*, look up, and locate the voice.

Dr. Kumar is not what I expect. He looks roughly my age and my height with an athletic build. Yes, he is Indian. That part I got right. I can tell by the surprised look on my wife's face that she thinks he is handsome.

Jocelyn helps me to my feet and I extend my hand to the young doctor. "Hi, Dr. Kumar. I'm Matthew Cavallo. Good to meet you."

"Likewise." We shake hands and he smiles. "Why don't you follow me back to my office and we can see what's troubling you."

I extend my arms, palms waist-high, and carefully step forward, right foot, left foot. Repeat. I notice that he lets me walk ahead of him. Not saying a word, I can feel his eyes watching me walk like a penguin. What is he looking for?

Dr. Kumar's office is all the way at the end of the hall. When we get to the door, he walks ahead and opens it. As I step into the room, I see that there is an examination table directly to the right and two chairs and his desk to the left. The walls are a soothing dark blue with his framed medical degrees hanging behind his mahogany desk.

I manage to maintain my penguin stride as we walk in, but, once there, I collapse into one of the chairs. Jocelyn sits down next to me. Dr. Kumar sits behind his mahogany desk. Jocelyn looks at me nervously, then at the doctor. Dr. Kumar sits back in his chair, crosses his hands, and looks at me.

"So, Matthew, Dr. Chalko says you are experiencing numbness in your lower extremities."

I take a deep breath. "Yeah. That's right."

"He's also having trouble going to the bathroom, Doctor," Jocelyn abruptly blurts out to make sure I don't forget to disclose that detail.

"Riiiiiiight," Dr. Kumar says. He pulls himself up in his chair, opens a desk drawer, and pulls out a white hospital gown. "Why don't you put on a Johnny, and we'll have a look at you."

He gets up from his desk, walks across the room, and pulls a curtain around the exam table. Then he gestures for me to step inside. Pulling myself up using the arms of the chair, I waddle behind the curtain. As I disrobe and put on the backless hospital gown, I hear Jocelyn tell Dr. Kumar about the various things she has observed about me during the week. Her nervousness has her babbling a mile a minute detailing all of my recent conditions with surprising accuracy. How does she do that?

I pull myself up on the table and call out, "Ready."

After a second, Dr. Kumar pulls the curtain open so Jocelyn can see the examination from her seat.

"Matthew, I want you to stand up. We're going to test your balance. Now close your eyes and stand straight."

I do as I am told. I close my eyes tight and stand as straight as possible. I maintain this position for a moment.

"Can I open my eyes now?"

"One moment, Matthew."

I am starting to wobble. I try to remain steady, but I feel myself wanting to topple down like a Jenga tower. Opening my eyes, I reach out my hand to balance myself on the examination table. I catch my breath. Never has standing been so demanding.

"Please do that again," is all the doctor says. "Only this time, could you please stand on one leg and with your arms spread out?"

What? Didn't he just see what happened? Okay, I'll amuse him. What the heck. Let's make fun of the wobbly boy. Once again, I stand as straight as I can. Then I spread my arms out and bend my leg. Before I can even close my eyes, I teeter over, grabbing the examination table on my way down. If these are tests that I am supposed to pass, this is definitely not going well.

"Okay, Matthew. Sit back down on the table and extend your legs toward me. Close your eyes and tell me if you feel anything."

The paper crinkles as I climb back up on the examination table. I can't feel the paper, though, I can only hear it. With my legs extended, I close my eyes and wait.

A minute passes. No one says a word. Isn't something supposed to be happening? Curious as to what is going on, I open my eyes a crack. The doctor is standing beside my outstretched legs, pricking them with a safety pin. I see the pin going in and out of my right leg. Then I see him do it to my left leg, too. But I don't feel the pin jabs at all. How can I not feel this?

He notices me looking. "Matthew, do you feel anything?"

I take a deep breath to calm myself down. "No," I say, wearily. "Not a thing."

"Look," he says. "Really concentrate and let me know if you feel anything."

He looks up and sees that I have my eyes open. "And close your eyes again," he says.

I pause for a second and try to really concentrate on my legs. I think that maybe somehow I can manufacture feeling through positive thought.

"I can feel it a little on my upper thigh," I venture. "I think. But I don't feel a thing as you get down past my knees."

"Riiiight," Dr. Kumar says. "Now I'm going to test your feet."

"Can I open my eyes?"

"Yes."

He takes out a key from his jacket pocket and runs it lengthwise down the sole of my foot. Ordinarily, I am very ticklish, so this should be driving me crazy, but, again, I don't feel a thing. Back and forth, forth and back. This is amazing. I usually burst out in hysterics even at the thought of someone touching my feet.

"Can you feel that?" he asks.

"No. I know it's there because I can see you do it, but I honestly can't feel it against my foot."

"Okay, close your eyes and lie down. I'm going to move your big toe up and down. Tell me which direction I am moving it."

"Okay."

The paper on the table crinkles as I pull myself around and lie down. I take a deep breath and try to relax. I am not sure what he wants me to do. After a bit he asks me about the toe movements.

"Which way is your toe facing now?"

I focus as hard as I can, waiting for him to do something. "Did you start yet?"

"Right."

Okay ... now that isn't his usual over-exaggerated riiiight. His voice is sharper than before. What the hell is going on here?

The curtain is open so Jocelyn can watch me as I fail all these tests. I haven't looked at her face until now. She is frozen in her chair. Her eyes are huge and filled with confusion and concern. I am not sure if she is still looking at me, or if her thoughts have started to run wild, taking her to some distant planet to process what she has just witnessed. Either way, her face tells me this is way more serious than either of us ever imagined.

"Okay, Matthew," the doctor says. "Put your clothes on, and we'll talk back at the desk."

Dr. Kumar steps back and draws back the curtain. At this point, Jocelyn steps inside. I am relieved to see her out of the chair and doing her best to appear calm, despite what she has just witnessed. She helps me put my pants and shoes on and then I squirm on the table and fasten my belt. When I look sadly into her eyes, she smiles back at me.

"It's going to be okay," she says, nodding her head to comfort me and herself at the same time.

Then she helps me to my feet. She holds me for a second as I stand up, and then we pull the curtain aside and go back to our seats to hear the diagnosis.

Dr. Kumar waits until we are seated. He leans forward in his chair. Crosses his hands on his mahogany desk. Then he takes a deep breath.

"Matthew, I believe you have a condition called Transverse Myelitis, which is a virus causing the inflammation of the spinal cord. This is causing you to lose the feeling to the lower extremities."

That's what Doctor Chalko said the other day! How come I couldn't remember that? I look over at Jocelyn and see that she has already written it down on a piece of paper.

Dr. Kumar continues, "This is just the initial diagnosis. We will know more when I get the results of the tests."

"Tests? What tests? What do you mean?"

He pauses again. "I want you to go check yourself into the ER at South Shore Hospital. I'm going to order a series of tests that will either confirm or disqualify my diagnosis. If it is TM, I need to put you on a steroid drip to dissolve the inflammation."

Wait.

What?

"The hospital? I've never been to a hospital in my life. Can't you just give me some medicine, and it'll go away?"

"I'm afraid not, Matthew. TM is generally caused by a viral infection. We need to run tests to see if you have a viral infection and find out how we can treat it."

I sit quietly for a few moments. I can feel Jocelyn looking at me.

"So when does he have to go there?" she asks.

"I'd like you to go there now. And you probably should pack a bag. I'll be honest with you. I think you'll be there for a couple of days, at least, depending on the results of the tests."

A couple of days! Man, what kind of virus is this?

~~~

We stand outside the sliding glass doors of the medical building, neither of us saying a word. The angry gray skies have opened up and rain is beating down on us.

Finally, Jocelyn breaks the silence. "I'm going to get the car, Matty. You stay here."

Her voice isn't strong, but it is clear. She pulls her denim jacket up over her head and races across the parking lot toward her car.

I stand still and watch the rain pelt the pavement.

Jocelyn pulls the car to the curb and I struggle to get down into it. The wipers are on overdrive, trying to deflect the pelting of rain on our windshield. Even in the car, we stay quiet, as I let Jocelyn handle the traffic. It isn't until we are almost home that I look over at her.

"Are you okay, baby?" I ask.

She is concentrating hard on the road. Visibility is very low.

"I think so," she says seriously, but then she let out a nervous laugh. "I just can't believe you have to go to the hospital, though."

"Me, either. Why are you laughing?"

It isn't a natural laugh. "I don't know. I can't help it."

I reach over and place my hand on the top of her thigh.

She forces a smile but her lips are slightly quivering. We pull into our driveway and sit quietly in the car for a few moments, watching the rain. I jitter with nicotine anxiety.

I can't fight the temptation any longer. "I hate to do this, but I need a smoke … bad."

"I don't care about that right now. Go ahead," she replies. "I'm going to pack you an overnight bag. Do you need anything?"

Need anything? What does one pack for the hospital? My wisecracking aside, I am still too much in shock. I shrug.

"I'm probably ready right now," I say. "I figure I'm going to walk out of there with a couple of those sweet Johnnys. Pretty attractive stuff, huh?"

Jocelyn laughs. A real laugh, this time, which makes me feel better. She steps out of the car and runs up to the house, covering her head with her purse, then opens the front door and ducks inside. She is way more worried than she is letting on, but she is putting on her bravest face for me.

I climb out of her car and penguin-walk over to my truck. I pull the door open and grab my pack of cigarettes from under the seat. To avoid the rain, and to light a smoke, I slide into the cab. Then I pull out my cell phone and begin systematically calling various people- my parents, my siblings, friends, and my office. Through brief calls and voicemail messages, I tell them all the same thing: I am on my way to the hospital to find out my fate.

Ten minutes and three cigarettes later, Jocelyn taps on my window. She is shielding herself with her blue denim jacket and carrying an overnight bag for me.

"You ready?"

"Yeah," I say, but really I just want to scream NO. "Let's go."

We climb back into the car and head to the hospital. Even though the drive is less than a mile, it seems to take forever. Jocelyn and I sit in silence until we arrive at the emergency room of South Shore Hospital.

The ER entrance is a large, automatic sliding glass door. Just inside are two maple-stained wooden desks, one on each side of the corridor. The sign on the desk on the left reads "Information," whereas the one on the right has no placard. Each is attended by hospital staff, an elderly volunteer behind the desk on the left, and a nurse on the right.

I don't want to walk in alone. Not now.

Standing just outside the door, I wait for Jocelyn as she parks the car. The rain pings on the steel roof above me. A couple of nurses are huddled around the corner, sneaking smokes. You think they'd know better. Then, again, maybe I should ask if they have an extra one for me. Before I have time to ask, however, I see Jocelyn running through the rain.

"You ready to go in?" she asks with a forced smile.

"As ready as I'll ever be. Let's go."

She puts her hand in mine, and we turn and walk through the sliding glass door and check in with the nurse at the reception desk to the right.

Chapter Ten - The ER

"Matthew Car-var-low?" a nurse calls out.

"Here," I shout, as if it is a roll call. "It's Ca-val-lo"

"Oh. Sorry." The ER nurse laughs.

Jocelyn helps me up and walks me into the exam room, just steps past the waiting room. I get up on the examining bench, and the nurse wraps a blood pressure cuff around my arm. My cell phone rings, but I send the call to voicemail. The automatic cuff constricts around my arm, beeps, and releases.

"120 over 80," she says, writing it on my chart. "You're fine. Open up and say, Ah."

As she is checking my temperature, my phone rings again.

"Sorry." I gargle on the thermometer stick and silence the ring again. "I guess people are worried about me."

"That's not such a bad thing, is it now?" She smiles and makes a few more notations on my chart. "Well, your vitals look good. They called ahead about your condition. Do you need a wheelchair?"

"No," I say quickly. "I can walk perfectly fine."

The nurse looks at me, incredulous.

Jocelyn jumps in. "I don't know about perfectly fine, but he can walk," she responds seriously.

The nurse looks at me again. "I'm getting mixed reports here," she says confused. "So tell me exactly what's going on with your legs? You're experiencing a loss of sensation? Correct?"

The novelty is wearing off. I mean, how many times do I have to repeat this? Shouldn't this be on a chart by now? My permanent record? I should just get it tattooed on my friggin' forehead.

Deep breath, Matt. They're here to help you.

I wind myself up again and recite my now scripted account of my current physical state.

I've been noticing that, over the last couple of days, I have a tendency to look all around and not at someone when I'm making my little speech. I mean, who wants to look someone in the face when you're talking about something so personal? But at the end of this version of the story, I pause and then look straight at the nurse.

She looks back at me for a couple of seconds. It seems like she wants to tell me something. Then a flicker goes through her eyes, as if she decides otherwise. "Did the doctor tell you what it might be?"

Knowing that I probably don't remember the name of the condition, Jocelyn jumps in to answer. "He said it might be Transverse Myelitis, but he wanted Matt to come and do some testing to make sure."

Again, the nurse looks like she is about to say something. "Okay. Well … um … I have all the information I need," she says. "Go ahead and have a seat in the waiting room. I'll get you in as soon as we have a bed for you."

I get up and turn to the door.

"Oh, and, Matthew?"

I turn to face her. "Yes?"

"Good luck."

Strange. Is that a good thing or a bad thing?

I smile at her.

"Thank you."

Slowly family members trickle in the waiting area of the ER and join Jocelyn and me. We all sit down and make small talk. Everyone wants to talk about something other than why we are actually here. Shortly into our riveting discussion of the weather, a male orderly calls out from a double door.

"Matthew Cavallo?"

"Here!"

Another roll call shout-out. You don't want to miss your turn around here and end up at the back of the line.

The orderly walks over to greet me. "Do you want me to get a wheelchair?" he asks.

"I don't think so."

"Well, it says here that you can't feel your feet or legs." His voice is too loud. "You might want to think about a wheelchair."

I wince at how loud his voice is.

"No, really, I can walk."

"Okay, just take it slow." Still too loud. "I don't want you falling on my watch."

I start to rise to my feet with Jocelyn holding me under one arm. She grabs her things and helps me over towards the door. That's when the orderly stops us.

"Sorry," he says, looking at Jocelyn. "You can't have any visitors with you until the doctor says its okay."

"But she's my wife!" I protest.

He must have heard that one before. "Sorry, no exceptions." He looks at me and then at Jocelyn. Jocelyn looks concerned.

"I'll be fine, baby," I say, trying to comfort her.

She looks deep into my eyes, and I can see the anxiety she is trying to hide.

"As soon as I have clearance, I'll bring you in to see him," the orderly assures her. He isn't talking so loudly now.

"Hopefully it's soon," I pipe in.

He smiles. "Are you sure you don't need a wheelchair, Mr. Cavallo?"

"I'll be fine. Let's go."

I start to head through the double doors when Jocelyn grabs me. "I love you, Matty,"

"Love you, too, baby. I'll be fine. Don't worry about me."

I hug her and give her a soft kiss on the mouth. I look deep into her eyes. I don't want to let on that I am scared of whatever is in store for me.

The orderly leads me to the ER staging area. I see several little rooms with their curtains closed, the nurses' station in the middle, and more beds parked around it. The nurses' station is a large circular desk in the middle of a big, square room.

Around the nurses' station are helpless patients in rolling beds with bags of fluids and beeping monitors. Most of the nurses are buzzing around, but one is playing solitaire at her computer. Ambulance drivers are rushing in and out, and a paramedic wearing a stethoscope is slowly pacing around the desk.

Organized chaos.

I try not to stare into the faces of the patients as I pass them, but it is like not looking at the people in a car crash. On those rolling beds is a lot of sadness and solitude.

The orderly puts me in a little corner room and hands me a Johnny and a plastic bag.

"Change into this. Leave on your underwear. Throw the rest into this bag. A nurse will be in shortly."

"Yes, sir," I salute.

I turn to face the bed. I drop the Johnny and the plastic bag on the bed, and then turn back around. And like that, he is gone. There is just flimsy sheet hanging in the doorway to shield me from every eye in the nurses' station. It is protecting my privacy, yet there is a small sliver open for me to see the comings and goings. Other than that, it is another one of those nondescript exam rooms.

On the wall is the same ubiquitous rack of outdated magazines. Even the hospital is a player in the outdated magazine scam.

I change into the Johnny leaving my boxers on underneath. And my socks.

"Mr. Cavallo?" a female voice calls from behind the curtain, "Can I come in?"

"Okay."

A young nurse pushes her way through the curtain. "Hi, Matthew. I'm here to take your vitals and put in your IV." She whips a digital thermometer out of her pocket and sticks it in my mouth. As she waits for it to register, she performs the other regular vital checks, pulse and blood pressure.

"Am I alive?" I joke.

"Yes, you're fine. I'm going to be putting in the IV. It's going to feel like a shot."

She is moving a little too fast for me.

"What's this for?" I squeak as she swabs my arm. "Are you giving me some kind of drip?"

"We're not using a drip. What I'm doing is inserting the IV so that it's easy access if the doctors need to put you on anything."

"So … it's just going to be sticking out of my arm?"

"For now, yes."

I cringe at the prospect of having a needle just sticking out of me, even though I am guessing that this is standard procedure. It is like I am now part of this big production line. Everyone knows their parts, but no one knows the master plan.

She quickly and expertly knots an elastic band around my left bicep. The veins in my lower arm begin to bulge. She puts my left hand in her left hand and turns it. A giant vein emerges on my wrist above my thumb. She runs her finger over this bulging vein like a jeweler inspecting a stone.

"This looks good," she says. She pulls a giant needle housed in a plastic case from her tray.

I turn my head.

"You're going to feel a little pinch."

I close my eyes and grit my teeth. Feeling the needle

pinch my wrist, I wince. "Ughhh," I groan through gritted teeth.

I feel the needle dive deep inside my vein.

"That's it," she says with a perky smile.

I turn and look at the IV in my wrist. It is a needle with a plastic tube. Connected to that plastic tube are two latex tubes with plastic stoppers. The nurse tapes the contraption tight to my forearm, leaving the latex tubes exposed. I work my wrist, turning it in a circular motion. The needle works its way deeper into my vein.

I wince again.

Then I look back up at the nurse. "So, I just have to stay with this thing stuck in me?"

"Yes. Is it comfortable, Matthew?"

"I guess it's as comfortable as a needle in a vein can be."

"Do you need anything else before I leave?"

"Yeah. Is there anything to eat around here? I'm absolutely starving."

She laughs again. "Dinner is over, but I'll see what I can do about bringing you a sandwich. Anything else?"

"A sandwich would be great. Maybe two, if at all possible."

"Okay, Matthew. A doctor will be with you shortly."

The nurse leaves and partially closes the curtain. With no TV to watch, I stare out into the nurses' station, hoping for either dramatic *ER* moments or comical *Scrubs* moments. To my disappointment, nothing at all is going on.

Moments later an anonymous male doctor walks into the room and shuts the curtain behind him.

"Hello, Matthew. I am an associate of Dr. Kumar. I spoke to him and he wanted me to check in on you."

"Okay."

I don't ask for his name. I notice he is wearing some sort of nametag on his coat, but I can't read it. He goes through the same battery of tests Dr. Kumar has already performed on me. Fine. I can deal with mindless repetition. Over and over. I just close my eyes and let him poke away. But then I hear the snap of a latex glove.

"Matthew, I need you to lower your underwear and roll on your side."

Oh, no, not again.

"Just roll over on your side."

I moan, but do as I am told. Is there even any relevance to these rectal exams? At least tell me the meaning. This random doctor just walks in here, does not even tell me his name, and yet goes full finger straight up my rectum. I usually like to at least know the name of the person that I am going to be that intimate with. Plus, Dr. Chalko already covered this. You'd think that there would be communication between the doctors. One of them says, "Hey, I did the dirty work. Here are the results. You guys can handle the rest."

I swallow hard. My parched throat tastes like a stale ashtray. Then it is over. The glove snaps as he takes it off. I am thinking these test should be more detailed. Not just a quick finger in the ass.

"Matthew, I'm sending you over for a CAT scan. An orderly will be here to get you shortly."

Great. First they probe my body. Now they probe my mind.

Chapter Eleven - Radiology

An orderly pushes my giant rolling hospital bed through the corridors as deftly as a grocery cart through a supermarket. Using my bed as a battering ram, he blows through some double doors and into a new section of the hospital. Man, this place is huge! Left on my own, I would be lost for days in this labyrinth. The corridors are empty. Desolate. I thought hospitals are always buzzing, like on *ER* and *Scrubs*. It is way too quiet here. A disinfected ghost town.

The orderly keeps wheeling me down the hall, not breaking a sweat. We approach a brown sign with white lettering. Radiology. The orderly slams the bed through the double doors under the sign.

I have seen CAT scans on TV shows and documentaries but never thought I would ever need one. Still no one has explained to me what they are actually looking for. Before I have a chance to think about that too much, the orderly cuts the wheels on the bed and parks me neatly up against a blank wall.

"Wait here," he says, as if I can move. "Someone will be out shortly."

"Hey, thanks."

But he is gone before my words come out.

My arm is itchy where the IV with the phantom tube is inserted. At least, I think it is the IV that is bothering me. I now realize that I am lying on an old wool blanket. For some reason, this starts to creep me out. Where else has this blanket been? Fortunately, a door opens and a nurse smiles as she walks over to me.

"Mr. Cavallo?"

"You got him." I answer.

"I am going to be taking you to your CAT scan." She

starts to unlock the wheels of the bed.

"Really? I thought I was already there."

"Almost." She expertly maneuvers the bed through another double door and into a brightly lit room. The CAT Scan machine looks like a six foot by six foot white plastic square with a giant circle cut out of the center so you can see through the machine. Extended from the empty circle is a rectangular plastic table with a sheet on it. On the opposite side of the room are tall glass windows. Through the glass, I see a man sitting at a desk. He comes out from behind the windows to assist the nurse.

"Matthew," the nurse says, "we're going to lift you onto this table."

"I can walk."

"Please, Matthew, just lie back and relax. We will assist you to the table."

Next they ask me to roll slightly to my side, as they lift me from the bed onto the table. It amazes me that this man and woman are able to pick up and move my 6'2", 215-pound body so easily.

Next they position me with my head inside the open circle of the square machine. Footsteps walk away. A door shuts. I am staring up into the room's florescent lights.

"Matthew?" This voice comes over an intercom.

"Yes?"

"Are you comfortable?"

"Well, probably as comfortable as I can be, given the situation."

"Good. Please lie completely still. This will only take a minute."

"Should I close my eyes?" I ask.

"It's up to you. It will not harm you, either way."

Harm me? That's a funny way of putting it.

"Okay." I decide to close my eyes and exercise that option.

"We're going to start now," he says.

I close my eyes as the machine begins to whirl. I take slow, gentle breaths and tune out the sound of the machine. I really need a smoke. I sense someone standing over me. I crack an eye and see a white-coated man.

"Matt, how are you doing?" he asks.

"I'm fine. Just waiting to start this procedure."

He laughs. "We're already finished. The nurse will be in momentarily to assist you."

I sit up. "Really? That wasn't bad at all."

A man and a woman are on each side of me. Again, I am lifted back onto the transport bed. The hospital's air conditioning has chilled my barely dressed body, so I squirm my way under the covers. The nurse wheels me out of the room and parks me against the wall.

"Matthew, someone will be by soon to escort you down to x-ray."

X-rays? No one told me I needed any x-rays. I wish someone would fill me in on what is going on here. First CAT Scan, now X-Rays. What's next?

But she is gone before I can protest. An orderly suddenly appears and looks over my chart, which is hanging from the foot of the bed. This is beginning to feel like a factory and I am a product on the assembly line.

"Are you ready to go, Matthew?"

"You're driving. I'll go wherever you want."

He smiles, and off we go. We maneuver through the dimly lit corridors for what seems like miles. A left, a right, another left, another right. I lie back and try counting the fluorescent lights above, but after fifteen, the novelty wears off. When I think I can't take it anymore, he brings the bed to an abrupt halt and parks me up against another wall in another nondescript hallway. He locks the wheels and is off like a shot.

I raise my head up and see another bed across the hall.

In it lies an elderly man whose body is frail and twisted. He looks toward me with his mouth wide open and utters some incomprehensible words. I just shake my head, signaling that I don't understand. Then I drop my head back down on the bed.

What's going on with me? I don't belong in here with the severely crippled. My legs are just a little numb. Or maybe I'm at the beginning stages of something as deforming as this old man has. Maybe he's not old at all, but the battle his body is going through has turned him into the man lying there across the hall. I don't want to look at him again.

I can see a room with glass windows and three nurses inside. One of the nurses emerges and checks my chart. This is getting to be a regular thing.

"Matthew?"

"Yeah?"

"I am going to be taking your chest x-rays. Do you think you can stand up?"

"Oh, yeah, no problem. Anything you need me to do."

She pushes my bed in front of a door, helps me stand up, and then leads me into a little room full of x-ray equipment.

"Matthew, I need you to remove your Johnny and stand facing the wall. Place your feet on the marks on the ground."

"Did you say remove my Johnny?"

I figure I better get clarification. As best I can remember, I only have my boxers on under there. I don't want to drop trousers then have her look at me and say "Now, what did you go and do that for?"

She is all business. "That's what I said."

I do as instructed and shuffle to the marks on the floor.

"Good. Now I'll adjust your chin rest. Once we have you in place, stand as still as possible until I tell you we're finished."

She is a bustle of activity.

"No problem. You're the boss."

As I press myself up against the wall, she steps back behind a heavy partition and takes a set of pictures. I listen to the machine whirr several times before she tells me I can sit down for a minute on a chair against another wall. She steps back into the room from behind the partition and instructs me that she wants to take one more set of x-rays to be safe. She has me get up again, and we repeat everything. After the second set, she helps me out of the door and back into the rolling bed. By now, I am beginning to get comfortable with letting people help me.

"Good job, Matthew. We need to x-ray your back now. Someone will be out in a minute to take care of you."

Another nurse emerges from the nurses' station. She drives my bed into a different room and places it directly next to a table.

"Matthew, lie still. We are going to move you over to the x-ray table."

"Okay."

Two nurses use the plastic board to shift me over to the x-ray table, which has a glass face with a huge light directly above it. The nurse tells me to lie still again as she leaves the room. I hear another machine whirring for a minute. Then she returns again, shifts me back to the bed, and parks me back out in the hall.

These tests are painless, but time consuming with a lot of waiting in between. A lot of chatter between hospital associates and a lot of taking pictures of my insides, yet no one has taken the time to explain to me exactly what they are looking for. If it is just a virus that I have, it seems like overkill with all these tests.

I have no concept of how long I've been here, but it feels like hours. Maybe Dr. Kumar is trying to finish all the tests tonight so I can go home. Either way, I wish someone would fill me in with what is going on around here.

Jocelyn is probably worried by now. She is supposed to come back and see me once I am settled. But that already feels like yesterday. All I know is that I really need to find the original nurse and that sandwich she promised me. I am starving!

Chapter Twelve - Admittance

After the x-rays, an orderly rolls me back to same ER staging room. No TV, no clock, no company. This place is a drag.

"Hello, Matthew. I brought you a sandwich."

Sweet Jesus! It is a miracle! There is my original nurse with sandwich in her hand.

"You are a life saver," I tell her. "I'm starving!"

"I think we can go out and get your wife now."

I smile, but barely acknowledge her as I rip into my sandwich. My first taste of hospital food is a dry tuna sandwich on white bread with a packet of mayo on the side. Although I'm not impressed, I tear into that sandwich as if it is my last meal. The mayo helps me choke it down.

Just as I finish inhaling the sandwich, Jocelyn comes walking toward me. She is carrying a bag from Subway.

I raise and point my wireless IV towards her like a gun as she walks in. "Move any closer and I'll shoot!"

"What is that thing?"

"It's my wireless IV, but I like to pretend it's either a super-secret spy gun or how Spiderman shoots his web."

It isn't that funny of a joke, but Jocelyn starts laughing uncontrollably. It is that weird, unnatural laugh that she had at Dr. Kumar's office. This is starting to freak me out.

"Is that a sandwich for me?" I say, my tummy still growling.

"Yes. Italian sub and a bag of chips. Your favorite. Your aunt and uncle brought it."

Just then a female doctor walks in. This is getting to be like the Grand Central Station.

"Matthew, I will be admitting you to the hospital this evening," she says.

Busy eating chips, I miss her name. To be truthful, I really don't care what her name is, considering the number of anonymous doctors, nurses, and orderlies that have already stopped by to check me and my strange condition out.

"Admitting me to the hospital?" I ask. "That's strange. I thought I was already in here."

"Yes, you are in the ER," she promptly replies. "But we had to do tests to see if you were going to be admitted to stay overnight. I also need to bring over the nurse to get your insurance information." She walks closer to my bed. "So ... tell me about your symptoms."

Here we go again. I look at Jocelyn.

"Right," I say. "Well, you know that feeling when you sit on something wrong and it falls asleep? That pins and needles feeling? Well it's like that, only it ranges from the waist all the way down to my toes. When I say from the waist down, I mean everything. I'm having trouble going to the bathroom and my genitals are not functioning normally. Dr. Kumar said he thinks it is Transverse Myelitis."

"I see, well I'm going to do some sensation tests."

She does the same tests that Dr. Kumar has already administered and I proudly fail each and every one of them...again.

~~~

The hospital room is standard. The walls are white and plain. A dry erase board on the wall at the foot of the bed gives me the name and phone extension of the nurse on duty. Above it hangs a small TV. There are also two stiff-looking chairs. To the right of the bed is a multi-colored curtain that separates the two beds. It is drawn, although there are no signs that I have a roommate. An IV pole stands behind the bed to the right, and to the left of the bed is a single small rectangular window with milky beveled glass.

The best feature of the room is the remote control. It basically controls my entire side of the room and allows me to radio out to the nurses' station. Being a gadget guy, this remote puts a little smile on my face in an otherwise depressing day.

Jocelyn pulls her chair over to my bed and reaches for my hand. I can see how tired she is by the look in her eyes, but I can also tell that she doesn't want to leave me. There is no clock in the room but it has to be close to midnight by this point and I know she needs to get some rest.

I get comfortable and turn on the TV. The speaker is poor quality and beeps periodically with hospital announcements or a nurse answering a call. Other than that, no complaints thus far.

Jocelyn sighs as she holds my free hand. "I really can't believe you're here."

"I know. I'm sorry."

"It's not your fault!" She rolls her eyes and looks around the room. We both burst out laughing.

"This is crazy, huh? I've never slept in a hospital room before."

"I don't want to leave you," she answers. "I can just sleep in this chair."

"That would be nice, baby, but I don't know if they're going to bring someone else in or how this whole deal works at night. Go home and get some rest and come over here tomorrow when you wake up. I'll be fine. I'm not going anywhere."

She laughs again. Her laugh is more normal this time.

"Okay. But make sure you call me if you need anything." She leans over and looks deep into my eyes.

"Don't worry about me. I'll be fine."

"I love you Matt." She kisses me and collects her purse and jacket.

"Love you, too, baby. See you tomorrow morning."

She reluctantly walks out the door, looking back at me in disbelief.

I know she wishes that she was staying here with me. Since we've been married, nearly three years ago, we've rarely spent a night apart. She is going to be worried and lonely tonight. I hate that I am only a mile away and can't sleep beside her.

Chapter Thirteen - Tuesday, May 24

Since Jocelyn's union benefits allow her to take up to five days off a year to tend to sick loved ones, she's taking the day off from work to sit with me at the hospital.

Today I wake up more helpless. Confined to a hospital bed with my will to move diminishing. The itching, irritating IV protruding from a vein in my hand still has no medicine attached to it, and I'm not getting any better on my own. You think they'd at least be medicating me. Why else would I have to endure the pain of this needle in my hand? I keep asking nurses and aides that question, and the answer is always the same. "Just in case." Just in case what?

I don't want to wear Jocelyn down with a hospital rant this early, though. She looks tired. She never really sleeps well when I'm not home. I think I make her feel safe. She's still in her workout clothes and glasses, with her hair pulled back into a ponytail. She doesn't typically wear her glasses outside the house, so I can tell she knows it's going to be a long day.

"The rain hasn't let up, huh?" I murmur.

"You should see it outside," she says. "It's a mess. I had a hard time driving over here."

"Ahh." I bat my eyes at her. "But that wasn't going to stop you now, was it?"

"You're a dork!" She rolls her eyes, and then she gets serious. "Did you have a good night's sleep?"

"No. I couldn't sleep at all. This place is a twenty-four-hour-a-day factory. There are people working all night. Machines beeping. Random intercom announcements. And nurses that come in and take your vital signs every couple of hours."

Just then, Dr. Kumar walks in. He is wearing a white

doctor's coat over his suit. Setting his briefcase on the floor, he walks over to my bed. Jocelyn is sitting to my left holding my hand, so he comes around to the right side.

"Good morning, Matthew. How are we feeling today?"

"I'm okay. Except for that whole no-feeling-in-my-legs thing."

"Riiiiiight." He picks up my chart and looks at it. "Well, we are going to start you on a three-day infusion of Solu-Medrol, which is an anti-inflammatory steroid. The Solu-Medrol should start to reduce the swelling in your spine, hopefully returning function to your legs. In the meantime, we are going to conduct an MRI of your back and neck."

"When will we know the results of the MRI?" Jocelyn asks.

"Possibly this afternoon, but they might not be ready until tomorrow morning," he tells her.

"So, I guess that means I am definitely in the hospital another night?" I already know the answer to my question.

"Yes, I am afraid so." He pauses. "Matthew, I have to go make my rounds now, but I will be in later to check on you again." He picks up his briefcase and walks out the door.

My chest tightens and a big ball of anxiety begins to build in the pit of my stomach. I need a smoke. It has been over twelve hours since I've had one, and I am definitely feeling the nicotine pangs. Without nicotine, how can I stifle my anxiety? *Shake it off, Matt.* These aren't the good old days when you could smoke in a hospital. Actually, is there any place socially acceptable to smoke anymore?

Just then the door opens and an orderly pokes his head in. Perfect timing.

"Good morning, sir. I'm here to take you to your MRI."

"Can she come with me?" I ask, pointing to Jocelyn.

"She can't go into the MRI room, but there's a waiting room if she wants to come for the walk."

Jocelyn sighs. "That's okay. I think I'll stay here and

wait. If your Mom or anyone else comes to visit, I don't want them to worry."

Come to think of it, I haven't heard from Mom at all since I've been in the hospital. Sure it's only been one night, but I am her first born. You'd think she would reach out to me in some way. But I guess I shouldn't be surprised. She never has dealt well with difficult situations.

~~~

The orderly pushes me and my bed through the double doors under the Radiology sign again and turns a different corner. Now I am in a square holding room with doors on three walls. The lighting is dim and yellow. In the background, I hear a constant, slight hum and a hiss that sounds like a pump motor. Over and over and over.

Chugga chugga psssst. Chugga chugga psssst.

"Matthew?" It is a female voice.

I twist myself up and look for the voice. "Yes?"

It is a middle-aged nurse poking her head out of the door to my right. "We're finishing up with another patient," she says. "We will be with you in a few minutes, so just hold tight."

"No problem. I can't think of anywhere else I have to be."

The door closes. I relax against the pillow and look up at the ceiling. A faint drilling sound overtakes the pump motor hum. The sound is reminiscent of a jack hammer outside the window of a city apartment.

A door opens and shuts. A bed is wheeled in front of me and in it lays a motionless young woman. I can't tell what afflicts her, but she looks like a teenager. Perhaps she has been in a car accident or something. I feel sorry for her, though, the way she is twisted up. She has something in a bad way. The nurse works to get her in a more comfortable position. She is not coherent in any way. Her mouth is open and drooling. A minute later, an orderly comes and whisks her away. I wish the best for her, even though I know that our paths will probably never cross again.

"Matthew, we're ready for you now."

As I am wheeled into the MRI room, I survey my new surroundings. To the right is a wall of glass with a computer console behind it. An Asian woman wearing glasses with round, black frames and a black pony tail is staring at the monitor, not making eye contact with me. A Caucasian man, six-feet tall with a good build, stands behind her, reviewing something on a clip board. Both are wearing white suits and look like they belong in some sort of radiation decontamination unit in a sci-fi movie.

As I scan to my left, I see the giant, white MRI machine. It looks like a giant plastic donut with a table extending out of the hole. The orderly pushes my bed alongside the table and lets the bed's rail down. The man in the radiation suit joins us. They push a plastic backer board under me, then the orderly and the radiation man lift me onto the table and pull the backer board out from under me. I feel so helpless not being able to make a simple movement on my own.

My head is placed into a padded half circle of plastic at the end of the table near the opening of the machine. Once in place, the man on my left completes the circle by lowering a half circle plastic mask over my face. The mask has three bars running up and down over my head. There is a mirror in the center of the mask. When I look into the mirror, I see it is trained on my feet.

"What am I supposed to be? Hannibal Lecter?"

The room is silent. Except for the constant hum of the MRI motor. Man, my jokes are just not landing. Don't these people realize how funny I am? I look up at the two florescent track lights at the entrance to the small tube. They are no more than inches above my head. I can't believe I am actually going to fit into such a small space.

A door behind me opens and closes. Footsteps shuffle up besides me. I am too fascinated by the opening of the MRI machine to notice.

"Matthew," I snap out of it and acknowledge the nurse that has walked up to me "would you like a pillow for under your legs?"

"Sure, why not? Hey, I'm not really going in that small little tube am I? I mean, I'm a pretty big guy."

She lifts my legs and puts a pillow underneath.

"Don't worry. You are going to do fine. I've seen much bigger people than you go in there. Just try not to think about it. Do you need a blanket or anything else to make you more comfortable?"

"No, I'll be fine," I answer, always obliging.

Radiation man walks around the table toward my head. He hands me a blue, rubber squeeze pump with a long rubber hose.

"Matthew, squeeze this if you need us to stop."

"Really? Cool."

Why would I need them to stop?

The table is cold, hard plastic. I lie there in my Hannibal Lecter cage, holding my rubber squeeze pump and waiting for someone to jump out and scream, "You're on Candid Camera!" Actually this whole experience feels like some cruel practical joke.

The machine continues to hum. Chugga chugga psssst. Chugga chugga psssst.

Then without notice the table begins to slide backwards into the donut hole. My shoulders scrape the side of the tube as I enter it. The wheels of the table click as they move me into place. The light dissipates as the table slides deeper into the MRI tube. Two tracks of dim fluorescent light, no more than three inches above my head, run the length of the tube. When I look at the mirror in my Hannibal Lecter cage, I can see my feet, but I am in too deep to see the light at the end of the tunnel. All of a sudden Radiation Man's voice comes over the loud speaker. He sounds like a trucker on a CB radio.

"Matthew, are you comfortable?"

"About as comfortable as I can be. This place is pretty tight," I reply in the most positive tone I can muster.

"Tight is good, the more still you can remain the faster we can finish. We are about to begin then. Take short breaths so you are not moving your chest. You will hear clicking sounds followed by a drilling sound. Remember, concentrate on your breathing and stay as still as possible."

"No problem."

Then it starts. The chugga chugga psssst is replaced by a noise I can best describe as that annoying tone that comes on when TV stations test the Emergency Broadcast System. But I don't let it get to me. I focus on staying still and breathing light.

Suddenly the noise stops for a moment, and all I can hear again is the chugga chugga psssst. I am starting to feel a tad disoriented. It feels like I have been in the tube at least ten minutes. Suddenly the wheels turn and the bed flows deeper into the tube. Sweat begins to trickle down my brow. I tell myself to just ignore it.

"Matthew." It is Radiation Man again. "We are ready for the next test. Keep it up. You're doing great."

The drilling begins again. This time is a higher-pitched, piercing sound. I feel like I am in Tron dodging laser beams. I brace myself to keep from flinching. My sweating increases as the claustrophobia sets in.

Focus on your breathing, Matt.

I remember back to a drama class I took in high school where I learned breathing techniques for meditation. *Inhale. Picture yourself somewhere else. Exhale. Picture a big hot air balloon soaring high above a green canyon.* Another ten minutes or so passes, then the noise stops again. The machine continues its old, familiar chugga chugga psssst.

Radiation Man is talking in my ear again.

"Matthew, you are doing great. We're going to move the table again for more pictures."

I swallow some stale air. The table clicks as it moves toward the end of the machine. Cool air blows on my toes, as if they have escaped the tube.

"Uhhh, I am feeling a bit disoriented in here. How much longer do I have to go?"

"Do you need to come out and take a break?"

"How long have I been in here?"

"Just over a half an hour. There are four different segments of your spine we are testing. We have completed the first two tests. Now if you can just stay still and not breathe so deeply, then maybe we can move this along a bit faster."

"Really? I've been moving? I'm sorry about that. I was focusing on not moving."

"Your head is twitching a bit. Every time you do, your spine moves, and we have to start over."

"Sorry. I'll try to be more aware of that."

"So, are we good?" he asks again. "Or do you need a break?"

Realizing that my questions are just making my confinement longer, I urge him to start it up again immediately. The drilling sound returns, louder and sharper than before. The track lighting above me seems closer now and the air is staler. Sweat puddles on my brow and my nose begins to itch. I quickly adjust myself.

"Matthew, stop twitching!" the voice bellows. "You need to stay still. We have to take these photos all over again."

But my little twitch has caused my sweaty boxer shorts to creep up my ass crack. I have manipulated myself into an uncomfortable wedgie. *Ignore it, Matt. Find that happy place.* The drilling continues. Although they've given me these squishy yellow ear plugs, they are not stopping the noise. I am losing my grip on the space-time continuum. My chest begins to tighten. I start taking big, gasping breaths. Then the machine stops.

I've been in this god-awful tube for at least an hour by now. My body is shaking slightly from the force of trying not to move. The itch on my nose is spreading across my cheeks, up to my forehead. The voice inside my head is taunting me to scratch it. My boxer shorts have turned into a thick, wet, cotton thong.

Breathe, Matt! Concentrate on breathing. This is all in your head.

Chugga chugga psssst. Chugga chugga psssst.

As if he is listening to my internal dialogue, Radiation Man's voice comes back on in the tube. The machine continues to hum.

"Okay, Matthew, we're going to pull you out of there. Stand by."

The table slides slowly out of the tube. As I emerge, I feel a burst of cool manufactured air. I squint through the bright light as my eyes readjust to normal room light. The voice is still with me. Is this the definition of God? Someone speaking to you in your head all the time?

"Okay, Matthew. A nurse will be in to insert an illuminating agent."

"Illuminating agent?" What the hell is that?

"We need to inject a dye into your IV. The dye will function as an illuminating agent for us to better see your organs. The dye will feel cool running through your veins. We will repeat the tests with the illuminating agent."

"Wait a minute. I have to go through all of the tests again?"

There is a pause.

"I'm afraid so. There are four different sections of your spine, and we need to take pictures of all of them."

Four different sections of my spine? My organs are about to be illuminated? What is going on here? Why don't I ask more questions? When is Rod Serling going to step out from behind the screen and tell me I'm in the Twilight Zone?

"I don't know if I am okay with all these tests."

"Matthew, we understand this has been difficult for you. You've been a trooper, though. Most people don't last an hour inside the MRI machine."

"Do you mean that I was in there for an hour already?"

"More like an hour and a half, but don't think about that. Typically, we would split these tests into two or three different sessions. In your case, however, the doctors need the data right away. I know this is a tremendous undertaking for you, but this is for your health." He pauses. "So, Matthew, are you with me? Do you think you can do it?"

I think about it for a second. If being in this tube is going to somehow help me get my legs back, then I will do it. I have no other choice. I also don't want to come back a second time. I want these tests done and done now!

"Get the illuminating agent. Let's get this over with." Can he hear the defeat in my voice?

"Good. Now you just relax."

A nurse comes out of somewhere pushing a little table and inserts a tube into my IV. In a few seconds, I feel the cool rush of a liquid coursing through my veins, air conditioning my insides. Then … back into the machine. The light from the room retreats and is replaced by the fluorescent of this plastic tomb. I am so hungry. My lunch is probably getting cold in my room. Jocelyn must be worried about me being gone so long.

The drilling starts again. I can't help but think of a recent *CSI* episode where one of the investigators is kidnapped and buried alive. The bad guys put him in a shallow grave and cover it with sand. The coffin is outfitted with a camera, a fan, and lights. When he regains consciousness, he starts feeling the top of the coffin with his hands, and then he begins kicking and screaming. He figures out where he is and what the situation is. Claustrophobia set in. His kicking and screaming turn on the lights and the camera in the coffin, which feeds the video to the CSI headquarters, where his team can only watch him struggle.

I feel like that guy. I can't take it anymore.

"Matthew, stop squirming, or we'll have to redo the test."

Hey! You come in here for five minutes and see how you like it! "I'm not moving," I answer with defiance in my voice.

A pause.

"Take shorter breaths then."

Here I am, struggling to stay alive, and this asshole tells me to take shorter breaths? *Walk a fucking mile in my shoes, pal.* Actually that kind of thinking isn't doing me any good. Concentrate on breathing. Go to a happy place. Never mind that the track lights are getting closer and closer as the ceiling caves in with each passing minute..

Chugga chugga psssst. Chugga chugga psssst.

"Do you need a break?" the radiologist asks.

Break? Yeah, I need to break the hell out of here.

I need to ….

… to get the feeling back in my legs, is what I need to do. I drop the blue squeeze ball so as not to press it inadvertently. *Forward! Press on!*

"No, I'm fine."

"Well," his voice sounds like he is frustrated, "you're moving around a lot. We're done with two tests. Come on, Matt. You can make it through the final two."

"Okay. Let's do it."

Okay, body, we're in lockdown mode.

Nobody moves.

Nobody makes a peep.

You got it?

Everybody play nice and nobody gets hurt. You hear me?

There is no rhythm, no comfort, no food.

I am going to suffocate in this tube.

If my legs were working, I would propel myself out of this damn donut and hit the floor running. Pay no attention to that crazy man in a hospital Johnny, frantically running through the halls, ladies and gentleman. He's only trying to escape that dreaded clicking machine.

"Okay, Matthew, we're almost there. Ten more minutes."

Ten more minutes!

Is that supposed to reassure me?

"We talked to the doctor. He doesn't need your lower lumbar region done again."

Great!

"Matt, try harder," This is a soft woman's voice.

Listen lady, you have no idea how hard I'm trying!

Suddenly the machine goes haywire. It is like an unholy electric symphony hitting its grand finale. I am forgetting that this test is to help me and my condition. These people are now the enemy. They are out to get me. I am sweating profusely again. I grit my teeth and push as hard as I can to control my body. Every cell of my organism is groaning under the effort and pushing myself to my physical limit.

To ...

the ...

breaking ...

And then the noise stops.

Just like that.

It's ... over.

The table moves me slowly out to normal light. The machine continues to hum.

Chugga chugga psssst. Chugga chugga psssst.

I look up. A man is standing over my bed and smiling.

"You did good, Matthew. Really good."

I recognize that voice. It is God. I mean Radiation Man, the radiologist.

He smiles down on me. "You're finished."

I feel finished.

I smile weakly. "Good. 'Cause after all that, I could really use a sandwich."

Chapter Fourteen - Some Troubling News

For the first time in my bed travels, I have a female orderly driving me. Maybe she will be more of a conversationalist. More sympathetic to my situation. But I am wrong. You can replace an orderly with a robot, and no one would know the difference. No matter what I say, she is not interested. I could say the bed is on fire or that she should be in the next *Sports Illustrated* swimsuit edition and she would probably still ignore me.

When we arrive back at my room, Emerson 484, I notice a big orange sticker on the outside of the door under the room number. I am the only one in my wing with an orange sticker. I should ask someone about that.

The orderly parks the bed at the door. I see Jocelyn sitting in the chairs next to my bed. I want to stand and run to her, but since I can't run, I just want to stand. Maybe a nice, short independent walk will burn some of this nervous energy I have trapped inside of me.

"I'm going to get a wheelchair to help you to the bed," the orderly says, breaking her vow of silence.

"Don't worry," I say. "I can take it from here."

"No, I can't let you do that," she says sternly. "You sit right there. I'll be right back."

Sit? After all that I have just been through, how can she expect me to just sit here? No way. The second she is out of sight, I swing my body to the side of the bed, slide down to the floor, and force myself up to my feet.

Just then the orderly returns with the wheelchair. She gasps as I stand up and penguin-walk into the room.

Determined to get to my bed before she has a chance to stop me, I shuffle my feet as fast as I can. Blood rushes to my head. I stumble a bit and reach to the wall for balance.

As I waddle across the room, I look to my left and notice I now have a roommate. He is knocked out. He seems to be about my age, but I can't make out much else.

Jocelyn springs from her seat and comes toward me.

"I can do it," I insist, waving her off.

After processing the situation, the frantic orderly finally pushes the transport bed out of the way and enters the room behind me. I pass my new roommate and make it to the edge of my bed without incident. Then I turn, lean up against it, look at the orderly and smile.

"I'm okay."

She looks relieved. I am happy to be walking again, and just as happy to finally get a rise out of her.

I pull myself up on the bed and pull my tray of food toward me. A small victory. Mission accomplished.

I settle back in my bed. "I told her I could do it. After being in that tube for over an hour, I had to get up and walk."

Jocelyn looks at me. "You were actually gone for three and a half hours," she murmurs.

"I was dying in there. I was in the MRI tube the whole time. I didn't think I was claustrophobic, but I don't know now."

I gaze down at my food. The lunch tray looks much better today. I have an unidentifiable pasta dish, another tuna sandwich, a salad, some fruit cocktail, a cup of green Jello, and a carton of apple juice. If I am going to consume stale food, I might as well order a filling amount. I start digging away at the meal.

I am halfway into my tuna sandwich, when an unfamiliar doctor enters the room. He is kind of a nerdy looking, with sandy brown hair and big round glasses. Probably in his early thirties.

"Hello, Matthew," he says in a nasally voice. "My name is Dr. Titleman, and I am the doctor for this floor."

"Hello, Dr. Titleman," I greet him as I chew. "My name

is Matthew, and I will be one of your patients on this floor."

Nothing. No response. He just keeps going with his routine.

"So," he starts poking me, "I understand you are having trouble going to the bathroom?"

I continue eating. I am used to random hospital staff poking at me by now. Plus, I am starving. I just want him check me out and leave.

Even though I don't answer, he continues on. "We're going insert a catheter to alleviate your bladder. Also, Dr. Kumar prescribed a steroid that we're going to administer through your IV."

I am so focused on my food that I'm really not paying attention to most of what he is saying. A quick glance at Jocelyn, though, and I can see she is a little nervous.

"Hey, whatever you guys need to do to get everything working again," I joke. "At this point, I'll try anything."

"Okay, then," he says, finishing the poking. "You rest up because you have a big day tomorrow."

"Okay, Dr. Titleman," I say between bites of fruit cocktail. "See you later."

He turns and makes his way to the other side of the curtain dividing the room. Now that it is drawn and cut the room in half, I also can't see who is coming or going.

"A catheter?" Jocelyn asks a minute later.

I laugh. "Well, I probably won't be able to feel it, anyways."

"I know." She pauses. "It's just the thought of it."

"Well, look at it this way," I respond. "It's just one less thing that I have to leave the bed and go walk and do."

"That's true." She smiles. "Way to look at the bright side."

I grin back at her.

"Want some Jello?" I ask, holding up a green glob.

She shakes her head.

I shovel the Jello into my mouth and drop my plastic spoon in the cup.

I lean back against my pillows. "Now, I think I'm going to take a little nap. I'm all worn out from the tests, and my internal clock is messed up, too."

"I am going to run to the cafeteria and pick up some lunch. Do you need anything?" Jocelyn asks.

"No, I'm okay." I am already drifting toward dreamland.

Jocelyn kisses my cheek but I am drifting further away. I just need some quiet time now.

~~~

"Wake up, Matthew."

My head is cloudy. I recognize the voice, but am not ready to open my eyes. "Oh. Hi, Shelly."

"Hello, Matthew."

Shelly is the day shift nurse assigned to me. She is probably in her late thirties, short, slightly overweight, with brown hair and a warm, welcoming smile. She has a motherly air about her. I can hear her moving items on her tray that she has pushed into the room. She is probably here to take my vitals.

"I'm going to put your catheter in now. You might feel a pinch."

My eyes shoot open. I bolt straight up in bed.

Catheter. Now that it is about to happen, I'm not in a joking mood.

Shelly looks like she is about to laugh from my expression, but she thinks better of it.

"Remember what Dr. Titleman said?"

"You mean he was a real doctor?" I reply. "I thought he was just some crazy man walking around the halls giving out insane recommendations."

Now she laughs.

"No, he's real. And you need a catheter."

"Oh, wow," I say, still coming to grips with the concept. "So ... um ... what do I do?"

"You don't do anything. I do it all. You just sit back and relax."

"Relax, huh? Hmm. Shelly, you know, I can't feel anything down there, but please ... be gentle."

"Oh I will. I promise."

I look at the bag and the tube lying on her tray. Then I sigh and nod my head. She tosses my blanket to the side and reaches under my gown.

She steps back. "Matthew, could you pull your boxers down for me?"

"Uh, yeah. I guess so." I wiggle around, pull my boxers down a bit, and turn my head away. This is getting strange. I do not want to see the tube entering my little buddy.

God, I don't want to see. But then again, I need to see. Someone is sticking something into my penis. Shouldn't I at least look to make sure they are doing it properly? After all, it is my penis. I have some long-term interest in making sure that it stays a functioning, able, body part.

Okay. Let's see what's going on down there.

I look down as she pulls the shaft of my penis straight up as far as it will go and is holds it there, like a little rubber Gumby. She then takes a pencil-tip-eraser-colored rubber tube and rolls it in what looks like lubrication. All one-handed! I guess she knows what she is doing.

Then she takes the tube and feeds it into my penis. I can't feel it, but the visual causes my back to lunge. She doesn't react to this. I am sure she is used to all sorts of namby-pamby reactions from men as she violates their most sacred possession. She must have figured out a long time ago that the best method is to keep plugging away. Pun intended.

She keeps feeding the tube further and further into my outstretched penis. The lubrication comes rolling back like a wave along the head as the tube enters deeper.

Okay, I think I've seen enough. I turn and look out the window. Drops of rain are hitting the glass and rolling down to the ledge.

"There you go!" Shelly steps back and snaps her latex gloves off. "That wasn't so bad, was it?"

"No, I didn't feel a thing. Unfortunately." But then I remember that Shelly just had my Johnson in her hand. I rethink this. "Well, maybe not unfortunately for you."

She laughs. "You're fresh! Okay, now I'm going to hook your IV up to the steroid drip that Dr. Kumar prescribed. But first I need to take some blood and your vitals."

"Ah, well. I expect no less. I mean, it's been almost forever since the last time."

She laughs again, and then turns serious as she extracts my blood, takes my vitals, and attaches my IV to a bag. Very professionally. It takes her about forty-five seconds.

Now, I officially look like a patient. My IV is all hooked up to a bag and I have a sack attached to my penis and hanging off the side of my bed. I am not comfortable at all. Not at all.

I stare at the catheter bag.

Yellow drops of urine begin to trickle down the tube. Fascinating.

This thing didn't take long to work, huh?

"Shelly," I say. "I'm feeling some pain."

"No problem, Matt," she replies. She leaves the room and is back in two seconds with a cup of water and a little pill. I swallow it thankfully.

Day two is coming to an end without any of my questions answered. I still can't walk. Everybody seems hush-hush about my condition. That MRI experience was brutal. And there is a lone orange sticker on the wall outside my room.

"Shelly" I say in my most pathetic voice. "I've been here almost twenty-four hours now. No one will tell me what's going on. And I still can't walk. To tell you the truth, I am starting to get a little scared."

She takes a dry towel and wipes my forehead.

"I wish I knew, Matt. I'd tell you. I swear. You just lie still and don't you worry. We're doing everything we can to get you on your feet again. I promise."

She fluffs my pillows and I lean back. With one line coming out of my wrist and another one out of my penis, I let the drug Shelly has just given me do its work.

I am in La-La Land before you could say ...la la.

~~~

The rain persists. I am slowly coming out of my drug induced nap. I look down toward the foot of the bed and see Jocelyn standing there.

My Dad and brother are also here.

They are talking to Dr. Kumar.

When did he get here?

Time to say something.

"Umm. Hello?"

The crowd turns its attention to me.

Dr. Kumar starts right in. "Matthew. Good. You are up. I was just about go over the results of your tests."

Finally. An explanation.

"Okay. What've you got for me?" I ask, bracing myself for anything.

"Your MRIs show lesions on your spine and brain. These types of lesions are consistent with three different conditions: Lyme disease, Sarcoidosis, or Multiple Sclerosis."

Multiple Sclerosis?

My Dad pulls his hat down tight over his eyes and starts fiddling with his thumbs. My brother's head sinks into his shoulders. He puts his hands over his face.

I'm sure Jocelyn is feeling it, too, but she pushes on. She turns to Dr. Kumar. "If you had to guess, Doctor, what would you say is the most probable cause?"

He takes another deep breath. Maybe he has emotions after all. "Riiiight. Well, it is hard to say for certain. I will need to conduct a spinal puncture on Matthew for a conclusive diagnosis."

A spinal puncture? What the hell is that?

"Spinal puncture?" I ask in a small voice.

He proceeds as if I am asking him if he takes sugar in his coffee. "You may have heard it referred to as a spinal tap. This is a necessary component to finding out what ails you. You see, Matthew, it is like a puzzle, and these tests are just pieces. Once we put them together, we will know what is affecting you and how to treat it. Without the research, we would just be guessing."

My next question is fairly obvious. "Does it hurt?"

"It is really quite standard. We numb the area on your back, insert the needle, and extract the spinal fluid. All you will feel is a little pressure near the injection area."

Insert a needle and extract spinal fluid.

Insert …

A needle …

And extract …

Is he serious?

I turn and look at Jocelyn. The horrified look on her face mirrors the feeling in my soul. Our eyes meet, but she quickly looks up at Dr Kumar. She doesn't want me to see the fear in her eyes.

"How long do we have to wait for those results?" she asks him.

"We should have all of the results back in about two

weeks."

Two weeks. I have to wait another two weeks?

Dr. Kumar looks around the room and into everyone's faces.

Silence.

My Dad nervously speaks up.

"Loretta, my sister, suffered from Multiple Sclerosis," he says. "She died about twenty years ago. She spent most of her adult life in a wheelchair. After she had the kids."

He continues to remember out loud the horrific disease that ravaged his sister. "At the end, she lost the ability to speak. All she could do was mumble."

My brother still has his head in his hands, staring at the hospital floor.

Jocelyn tries to shift the focus off of MS. "What was the third one you mentioned, Dr. Kumar?" she asks.

"Sarcoidosis. This is a multi-system disorder that generally affects the lungs. The disease creates abnormal masses in certain organs that are formed from abnormal white blood cells."

I already know in my heart that this Sarcoidosis is a long shot. My lungs are fine. It's my legs, penis, and everything else south of my waist that has lost life.

The room is silent.

Someone say something.

Dr. Kumar must sense that everyone is processing the magnitude of what he has just said, so he proceeds. "As I said before, the lab tests generally take two to three weeks to process. I am going to schedule an appointment with Matthew around the second week of June. I also need to look at the film. As the pieces of the puzzle come together, we'll know which direction to go with treatment."

We are still in May. Am I supposed to just wait in limbo until then?

"That seems like a long time to wait," I say.

"Well, the best thing you can do is rest." He takes a step backward. "I have to make my rounds now, but I will be back tomorrow morning to conduct the procedure."

"Thank you, Dr. Kumar," I say.

He smiles and excuses himself from the room.

I can see that my Dad is becoming increasingly uncomfortable with his thoughts and this hospital visit. He makes his way to the side of my bed and puts his hand on my shoulder.

"I have to get out of here, pal. I have to go see a guy about a job."

Nice cover, Dad. But I know he is going to go home to break the news to Mom. They will probably both start blaming themselves, and eventually each other, for giving me this disease, whichever one of the three it is. They will both immediately assume the worst case scenario and have me confined to a wheelchair for life by lunchtime. They aren't exactly glass-half-full people. I am just thankful that their pity party isn't going to be played out in front of me. For now anyway. I need people around me right now that are going to be strong because I am not sure how much longer I can keep up my strength.

"Okay, Dad. Thanks for coming by."

My brother steps forward and offers me a high five. "I've got to head out, too, bro."

No, he definitely is not the pillar of strength I need now, either.

"Well, thanks for coming by."

They kiss me and head out the door. It is just as well that they make a quick exit.

Jocelyn comes to the bed and motions for me to scoot over. She lies down next to me and we stare up at the TV. There are too many emotions running through our heads.

Suddenly, I remember something important.

"Hey! Did my dinner tray come yet?"

She laughs. "No, it's not here yet. The woman came when you were with Dr. Kumar, and one of the nurses told her to come back in a minute. I'll see if I can track her down."

"Good. I could really use some food."

Chapter Fifteen - Wednesday, May 25

I open my eyes. I am on my back with my head facing the window. It is morning, but the sky is still an ominous gray. I turn my head and see Jocelyn sitting quietly beside my bed. The red and blue of her Arizona Wildcat sweatshirt mixes with the morning gray to create a purple aura around her. I rub the sleep out of my eyes and reach out to her.

She sits down on the bed, wraps her arms around my shoulders, and kisses me gently on my lips. "Good morning."

I point to the curtain dividing my bed and my roommate's half of the room. "Is he asleep?" I mouth.

She gets off the bed and creeps around the corner curtain and looks him up and down. Then she comes back. "He's really passed out," she whispers. "What do you think is wrong with him?"

"I have no idea," I say, "but he hasn't moved all night. And there's that orange sticker on our door. It's the only one in the hall. It has to be for him, right?"

Jocelyn shrugs her shoulders. She isn't very interested, but I think there is a definite orange sticker conspiracy. I want to get to the bottom of it. To escape my thoughts about my own fate, I come up with a 101 possible meanings for the mystery sticker.

"Let's not talk about him," she says. "How'd you sleep last night?"

I yawn. "I haven't really slept at all," I answer. "I can't get comfortable sleeping on my back. This stupid IV needle keeps digging into me, and it never really gets dark or quiet at night around here. I think I am actually going to close my eyes for a few more minutes. Do you mind?"

Shelly walks in before Jocelyn has a chance to answer. "Good morning!" she chirps. "Time to get you ready for your

MRI."

I look at Jocelyn, who looks back at me. We are both confused.

"Wait a second," I say. "What MRI? I just had one yesterday."

Shelly looks down at her clipboard. "Your chart says you have an MRI this morning."

And just like that, whatever calm I am feeling vanishes.

"No, no, no! The chart's wrong. I have a spinal tap this morning!"

She taps the chart with her finger. "It says right here you are going for more tests."

"Wait, a minute. Shelly, I already did the MRI yesterday. This has to be a mistake. Dr. Kumar didn't say anything about another MRI. I have my spinal tap today." I blink my eyes, remembering the claustrophobia. "I can't go in that stupid tube again!"

"Oh. It says here that Dr. Titleman ordered the MRI."

I shake my head vigorously. At least that part of me moves. "Excuse me, but who in the hell does Dr. Titleman think he is? He certainly isn't my doctor. He hasn't been doing any of my procedures!" I am screaming now. "All I know about him is he walked in here one night when I was groggy, introduced himself, had you stick a tube in my dick, and walked out. Thanks, but no thanks. There is no way I am going to go do any fucking tests for Dr. Titleman!"

Shelly's face drops as her prize patient turns into a flagrant asshole. "Matt," she says, "I'm sorry, but they're coming here to take you down. Right now."

"They are not taking me anywhere. Shelly, I'm not going to do it. I can't."

I look helplessly at Jocelyn. She turns to Shelly.

"Is there any way he can get a sedative or something?" she asks.

"I don't need drugs! I'm not going back in there!" I

scream.

Shelly looks at me. When she sees that I am not going to budge, she does the best thing she can do at this moment. She walks out of the room.

"Matty," Jocelyn says, "I know you had a bad experience yesterday, baby, but you have to do this. These people are here to help you."

"Joci, I can't do it. I can't go back in that damn tube. I can't! I swear I can't!"

Just then Shelly hurries back in, big white pill in hand.

I fold my arms and scrunch my face like a four-year-old in the middle of a tantrum. "I don't need that!"

"Take it, Matt," Jocelyn urges.

Like a petulant child, I grab the pill, shove it in my mouth, and swallow hard.

Shelly flips through my chart, and then looks me dead in the eyes. "Matt, I really have no control over where you are supposed to be or what you have to do. I'm just doing my job. All I know is that there's an MRI on your chart this morning."

I sigh. How can I possibly yell at Shelly? "I know, I know," I mumble. "I'm sorry, Shelly. I don't mean to shoot the messenger." I pull the blanket tighter around me. "It's just ... you know ... I've been poked and prodded enough since I've been here. And I still don't know what is wrong with me. I'm tired of being in the dark."

"I know, I know," she says. "I understand how you feel. You're doing a great job, Matt. Just hang in there." Then she walks out of the room again.

Oh, God, what an asshole I am. She is the only one here that actually laughs at my jokes. I feel about two inches tall. But, still, what is up with Dr. Titleman? Who does he think he is, ordering tests for me?

He is probably trying to rack up my insurance bill. How much is this extra MRI going to cost anyway? I am not even sure what our insurance covers. I have a friggin' mortgage to think about, and now I'm going to have to worry about how to pay hospital bills, too? That's if I still have job after all of this. Actually, with this bill, I'll probably need two stinking jobs. Thanks, but no fucking thanks.

I cross my arms and prepare to dig in my heels. But the drug is starting to take effect. I am losing my will to fight. Then I look at Jocelyn and see the look in her eyes.

"Baby, if he wants you to go, just go."

"But I was there yesterday." I am feeling mildly sedated.

"It doesn't matter," she says. "That's what they need you to do. So do it, and let's get you better. Stop fighting the people trying to help you."

There she goes again. Making sense.

Shelly comes back into the room. She looks like she has fought for me, but lost. "Dr. Kumar prescribed the MRI's and Dr. Titleman was the one who wrote the order," she tells me. "They want to do an MRI of your neck and brain. Those were not done before."

I retreat. I feel bad about how I behaved.

"Shelly, I'm sorry about earlier. I didn't mean to be such a jerk. I just didn't understand who gave Dr. Titleman the right to order me around."

The look on her face is that of a woman with a short memory. This is her job. She's already moved on. "Matt," she says in her professional voice, "you've been through a lot. I know this is a scary experience for you. I completely understand where you are coming from. Just understand, we are here to help you. We are a team of people who are trying to get you back on your feet."

She is right.

"I know ... I know ... I'm sorry ... I'm just scared." I smooth out my blanket. A renewed confidence comes over me. "Well," I finally say, "let's go take some pictures of my brain, shall we?"

The sedative has now rushed a warm calm over my body and mind.

The orderly arrives and parks the bed outside. She has a wheelchair this time. They won't let me walk to the door and get on the bed. Without a word, Shelly and the orderly move me from the bed to the wheelchair and then lay me on the rolling bed in the hall. And so begins another long journey through the endless corridors and elevators to my torture chamber.

~~~

Here I am again. Parked in the hall outside the MRI room, listening to the clicks and whirls of the machine. It is like Old Home Week.

Chugga chugga Psssst. Chugga chugga Psssst.

Oh, well.

Alone again.

Man versus machine.

Only this time, I am sedated. My will to fight is gone.

A nurse comes out of the room and leans over me. "Matthew, there are a few patients ahead of you," she says. "There is another option. If you're interested?"

"Another option?"

"We have a mobile MRI unit. It's on the other side of the hospital. They can see you now if you want to go over there?"

This is a kind of no-brainer. "Sure, I'll give it a try if it will speed this process up."

The elevator opens and I am off on a new adventure.

We zoom down a corridor with floor-to-ceiling windows. It is raining buckets outside. Maybe I did pick a good week to be hospital-bound, after all. I see a dark blue RV parked on the other side of the windows, and at the end of the corridor is a big metal garage door with two guys standing in front of it. I assume they are the radiologists.

"Hello, Matthew, thanks for coming down here."

What is this? A country club?

"Hey, thanks for having me," I say, continuing the forced civility.

"Well," one guy says, "just relax, okay? We'll take care of you. What we need to do now is to get you inside the unit. We're going to roll you into this elevator and then raise you up onto the unit's platform."

"Okay," I say. "Am I gonna get rained on?" I am skeptical of the process.

"No," the other guy answers. "It's all covered."

On second thought, I haven't showered since I entered the hospital. Maybe a splash of rain wouldn't be so bad. But, as promised, I am transported onto the lift and up to the mobile unit without getting a drop of rain on me.

The inside of the unit looks a lot like the MRI room. There is a glass panel to the right, behind are the computers. To the left is the big MRI tube, which I see now is manufactured by GE.

This staff here seems more relaxed.

Or maybe it is just the sedative?

"Matthew, we are going to release the locks on your bed and lift you on to the table. Can you roll to the right?"

"I think so." I roll slightly to the right and feel them shove a plastic board under me. Once secure, I roll back, and they lift me up and onto the MRI table and place my head in the familiar Hannibal Lecter confines.

I look straight up, focusing on the ceiling.

No twitching this time.

Short breaths.

Happy place.

"Would you like a pillow for your legs?"

"Sure," I say.

"What about some music?"

Man, is this the spa part of the hospital? How come no one told me about this before? Music?

"Got any Tom Petty?" I ask.

"Excellent selection, sir. We have his *Greatest Hits*. We'll just put the headphones on you and push you back into the machine."

"Let's rock," I say.

Headphones are slipped over my ears and I am handed the rubber emergency squeeze pump.

"Just squeeze this if you need to stop."

The table clicks as it pushes me deep into the donut hole. The track lights above me are already on. And then the opening strains to "Break Down" come through my headphones.

I don't have the strength to fight it this time. I need to remain as still as possible. So I never have to do this again.

The music stops.

"Matthew? Are you comfortable?" The voice comes through my headphones.

"Pretty much," I answer.

"Good. We are about to begin. It's the same drill as the last time. Remember, concentrate on your breathing and stay as still as possible."

"No problem."

It's all right if you love me. It's all right if you don't.

Tom Petty's nasally vocals fill up my head.

I don't have the urge to squirm this time. The sedative is working. I can feel a tingling sensation in my fingers, and then my whole body begins to mellow out. I start to drift off, but realize I need to stay awake.

Stay focused.

Chugga chugga psssst. Chugga chugga psssst.

The familiar sound rings in my ear, followed by the Emergency Broadcast System drill sound. The machine noises are muffled by the headphones and Tom Petty. But I can still hear them faintly.

Stay focused.

Chugga chugga psssst. Chugga chugga psssst.

~~~

"Matthew?"

Chugga chugga psssst.

"...Matthew?"

The men in white masks are over me again.

"What? What happened?"

"Nothing. We're finished."

"Finished? What about the illuminating agent?"

"Already taken care of."

I am puzzled. Where am I? I can feel a breeze on my arms. Whoa! I don't remember being pulled out of the tube. "Really?" I ask.

"Yeah. You don't remember?"

"No. Not really," I say.

"We pulled you out and you asked if you were staying still and doing a good job."

"Was I? I mean, did I?"

"Yeah. You were perfect," he says. "Now, let's get you over into this bed."

"I think I must have dozed off. How long was I in there?"

"In total?" the radiologist asks.

"Yeah."

"About an hour and twenty minutes."

"Man, those are some good drugs."

Chapter Sixteen - The Spinal Tap

"Dad really wanted to be here, but he has a very important business meeting."

A familiar voice is speaking just a little louder than a whisper. The voice seems far away. It echoes, as if I am lying at the bottom of a deep well.

"And Michael has band practice today, and Nicole is at work, but they should be here later. But you know how busy they always are." It is my Mom.

Then I hear another voice.

"I wouldn't worry, Rosie. Matt knows they would be here if they could."

Ahh, that is Jocelyn. Definitely Jocelyn. I am drawn to the sound of their conversation, but not ready to open my eyes quite yet. Instead, I just listen and float between various states of consciousness.

"Look at him lying there," Mom cries out. "This just isn't like him. He is such an ox. I don't remember him ever being injured or sick. Ever. He had allergies and asthma, but that was all. " Her voice is becoming shaky. "I just can't stand—" She stops, and I hear a rustling sound, then the screech of a chair being dragged across the linoleum floor.

"I just can't...." Her voice splinters. "I just can't stand seeing him like this," she wails. She sounds like she has just identified my cold, dead body at the morgue.

Even with my eyes closed I can see the tears.

At this point Jocelyn probably has her arm around her, comforting her. Mom is sniffling like she has a really bad cold. "What if he's never the same again?" she asks.

"Rosie," I hear Jocelyn say quietly, "we have to think positively. He is going to be okay."

There is a long pause. Then I hear Mom again,

whispering, "What if he was exposed to radiation in the Navy?" Her voice increases in volume. "I've heard stories of that happening, you know. Or it could have been all those allergy shots he received a child. I never should've listened to those doctors. The drug companies are always trying to poison people."

She pauses.

"What if it turns out to be MS? I wasn't going to marry Peter because of how Loretta was. I was afraid something like this would happen to one of my kids. The doctors told me it wasn't genetic. If only I hadn't married Peter. Oh, God, THIS ... IS ... ALL ... MY ... FAULT." By now she is choking on her tears.

"What did I do?" She is panting gasping for breath. "WHAT DID I DO?" The emotional volcano has erupted.

Jocelyn tries comforting her. "Rosie, he's going to be okay. We have to think positively. For Matt's sake."

But there's no comforting Mom when she's like this. Believe me, I know. It is upsetting for me to lie here, listening to her talk about me like this. How did all of this turn into a pity party for her? I'm the sick one, right? If she hadn't married my Dad, I would have never been born. I have to stop the drama.

I open my eyes. Mom and Jocelyn are sitting in the chairs against the wall at the foot of my bed. Mom's baggy maroon sweater covers her arms, and her head is buried in her hands, with her stringy, dyed brown hair hanging over her fingers.

"Hi, guys." I yawn, stretching my arms over my head.

"Oh ... hi, Matt!" Mom pushes herself away from Jocelyn and wipes her eyes. Her eyes are puffy and irritated and her makeup has run down her face.

"Has Dr, Kumar been by yet?" I say diverting attention away from the breakdown.

"Not yet." Jocelyn reports. "But Shelly was in here a

little bit ago and said he would be here soon for the spinal tap."

As if by magic, a nurse I have never seen before wheels a cart into the room. She is in her forties, with brownish-blonde hair, blue tinted glasses, and wearing a set of green scrubs with yellow floral print pants. Set on top of the cart is a shiny metal tray piled high with plastic tubes, syringes, and several different epidural needles ranging in size from big to huge. One needle looks as if it could go in my back and out my chest.

Maybe I should rethink this whole spinal tap thing. Not that I have a choice. It isn't exactly a voluntary procedure.

"Hi, Matthew," the nurse says as she parks the cart at the foot of my bed. She probably doesn't want me focusing on that tray of medieval torture devices. "My name is Terry, and I am going to be assisting Dr. Kumar today. Have you had an epidural procedure before?"

"Uh, that would be a negative," I answer. "But, you know, I've heard a lot about it. Good things, of course."

No response. My humor seems to be lost on everyone at the hospital. Except Shelly. I wish she was here for this.

Terry starts fussing with the curtain around my bed. But Jocelyn, my Mom, and I cannot stop staring at the humongous needles on the tray.

Just then, Dr. Kumar arrives, wearing the standard white doctor's coat and carrying his briefcase, like it is just another day. Shelly bubbles in right behind him. She looks happy, like she is totally over my earlier outburst. What a relief. Seeing Shelly smile at me makes the impending procedure easier to stomach.

Dr. Kumar greets Jocelyn and my Mom. I think he says hi to me, too, but, to tell you the truth, I still can't take my eyes off those monster needles. I think Mom feels the same way. She keeps looking over at the tray, then back at me. Her eyes look strange.

At least Jocelyn is holding it together. She is looking at Dr. Kumar calmly, waiting for what is to come. Maybe she is trying to keep herself from looking at the needles.

As usual, Dr. Kumar gets right to the point. "Matthew, are you ready to begin?"

"I think so. Can my Mom and wife stay?"

"Riiiight," He pauses to think. "I would rather they not stay."

"That's okay," Jocelyn says. She turns to Mom and nudges her toward the door. "Rosie, we can sit in the waiting room down the hall. I have to call and check in with work, okay?"

Mom nods, as if she is waking up from a dream, and walks back to my bed, hugs me tight, and kisses my cheek.

She pulls away, her face worn with worry.

As Mom pulls back, Jocelyn steps forward and throws her arms around me. "You'll do just fine." She gives me a hard hug. "I know it." She kisses me firmly on the lips. "I love my Matty friend."

"Love you, too, baby"

The medical staff takes this as a cue to get started. I hear the tray wheels squeak as my Mom and Jocelyn head out of the room. Shelly springs into action and pulls my bedside curtain all the way closed. Good thing my roommate is all doped up. I do not want to worry about strangers witnessing whatever is going to happen to me now.

"Are we going to do this in here?" I ask. "I mean, there isn't a spinal tap room or torture chamber?"

"Riiiight." Dr. Kumar isn't quite getting the joke. "This will be fine, Matthew."

He is taking inventory of the tray. Once he is sure he has each instrument required for the procedure, he addresses me again. "Matthew, we need to get you to sit up. Shelly can you help?"

"Sure." She races to my left side and lifts my legs over the left side of the bed, twisting my torso into a sitting position. With all of the tubes I am hooked up to, it is quite an endeavor.

Once I am in position, Dr. Kumar says, "Good. Now place your elbows on the table in front of you and arch your back out towards me."

I put my elbows square on the table and rest my face in the palms of my hands. I am looking directly at the window, which is still streaked with rain. All I can see is a gray, rainy day. Is this rain ever going to end? Maybe the world crying for me.

"Shelly," the doctor says, "could you untie his Johnny? I need unobstructed access to his back."

She reaches around and unties my hospital gown. "Don't worry Matthew. You're going to do great."

Dr. Kumar comes around from behind the bed to face me. "Don't worry, Matthew. This is a common procedure. It is a critical component in us being able to arrive at the correct clinical diagnosis. It is fairly uncomfortable, but I will keep you informed of each step. Do you have any questions for me before we begin?"

"No. I'm ready to get this over with."

"Okay, then. Terry, can you place the dressing on Matthew's back?"

I turn my head to the right. Terry has a back-sized, rectangular sheet of green flimsy plastic with adhesive tape along the four sides. There is a small rectangular hole in the middle. I can feel the adhesive taped being fixed to my back.

"Good," says Dr. Kumar. "Now, Matthew, we are just going to rub iodine on your back to disinfect the skin and prevent infection."

Terry and Dr. Kumar are behind me talking to each other, and Shelly is standing in front of me eyeing their progress and awaiting orders.

I feel a cool liquid being rubbed over the middle of my back.

"Good," Dr. Kumar says. "Now we are ready to proceed. Matthew, I am going to inject a local anesthetic into the lower lumbar region of your back. You will feel this needle. Then you will feel numbness in the area. Let me know when you are completely numb."

I feel the bed sink a bit as he climbs on the bed to reach me. Then I feel a cool hand on my back. He uses his fingers to elevate a patch of skin. The needle pricks the elevated patch. I flinch, gritting my teeth. I feel something entering my back.

"Ughh."

A minute or two passes as the medical team waits for the drug to take effect. Dr. Kumar and Terry are strategizing behind me, but I can't understand what they are saying. Shelly stands in front of me, comforting me with her smile. I turn my eyes and watch the rain beat against the window. The window is high in the wall, so all I can see of the world outside is a thick storm cloud layer.

I hear Dr. Kumar again. "Now, Matthew, do you have any feeling in your lower back?"

"I'm not sure."

Doesn't he remember what I am in here for? Hello? How can I possibly know if the middle of my back is numb unless someone is hitting me or something?

"It's probably ready if you want to try," I say.

"Okay. You are going to feel pressure, which is normal. It may not feel comfortable, but there should not be any pain."

Yeah, right.

"If you start to feel pain in any way, tell me and I will stop."

I brace myself for the big, big needle. "Okay. Let's do this!"

I am not kidding. I really want to get this thing over with. I have had my fill of this place. I have been poked and prodded in here for three long days. I just want to go home, sleep in my own bed, and cuddle with my Jocelyn.

"I'm here if you need anything," Shelly says. Her voice makes me feel better. She is so warm, so comforting, so motherly. Even after our incident earlier.

Just then I feel some pressure in my lower back. The pressure comes quick and hard. And it hurts like a son of bitch. Didn't Dr. Kumar say there wasn't going to be pain? Shit!

I close my eyes and swallow hard. This isn't going to be easy. It feels like a small sword is being pushed slowly into my back.

I open my eyes and stare sadly at Shelly. She smiles back. I try to focus my attention on the rain hitting the window. The pressure increases. Blood is rushing to my brain. I keep hearing this strange metallic ringing in my ears.

Then the pressure stops. There is muffled conversation going on behind the bed. I can hear movement. Clanging sounds on the metallic tray.

A minute or two passes. Shelly looks concerned. I am fine. This doesn't hurt nearly as much as I thought.

Then it is back. With a vengeance. The pressure returns. A sharp pain shoots up my back into the base of my neck. Tension begins to mount in my lower back near my waist. I wriggle my bottom a bit, trying to get more comfortable.

"Matthew, please stay still. We've had a small complication."

Complication? What kind of complication? It has been at least ten minutes by now, I thought we were almost done.

Another couple minutes pass.

The pressure is wearing on me. It feels like someone is piling bricks on my back. I am beginning to feel faint. Sweat begins to bead on my forehead. The pain is unbearable. I have to say something.

"Dr. Kumar, this is really uncomfortable."

"Sorry, Matthew, but this is not going as expected."

I turn my head and look at Shelly again. Her trademark smile has turned into a stricken look of concern.

The pressure is growing increasingly worse. I am suddenly short of breath. Sitting, leaning with my elbows on the table while arching my back is becoming almost intolerable. I adjust my elbows a bit, searching for a more comfortable spot.

"Matthew, hold still."

What can I do? I need to find a more comfortable position, but I am frozen stiff by a gigantic needle poking deeper and deeper into my spine. If I move the wrong way, will I be paralyzed for life?

I really have to start asking more questions before I let them do these things to me.

Sweat is raining down my face and stinging my eyes. I am burning up. A strange taste floods my mouth. The ringing in my ears grows stronger. The pressure has spread from my lower back up my spine. My entire back and neck feel severely bruised.

Finally, Dr. Kumar breaks the silence. "Matthew, we have a problem."

"WHAT?"

"You have a calcification in the ligaments at the spot of entry. I have been unable to get all the way through to the spinal cord. I tried a smaller needle to make the process as painless as possible, but I had to switch to a bigger needle. I knew the level of discomfort would increase, but we had to get through this."

"Okay. So, are you finished now?"

"Unfortunately, we were unable to gain access from this point of entry. I tried to manipulate the needle through the calcification, but even the bigger needle was unable to get through. Unfortunately, we must proceed with the worst case scenario. A double puncture."

"A double puncture?" I am perplexed. "A double puncture? I thought this was over. You mean you have to go in again?"

"Yes, but in a different spot further up your spine," Dr. Kumar continues in his matter-of-fact voice. I can't see him, but I can tell he is serious. He is always serious. "We will numb the new area, but this is a more sensitive area than the first entry."

What does he want me to say? What else can I do? It's not as if we can take a break. I don't want to drag this thing out any longer than necessary. Now is the time. I take a deep breath and exhale.

"Let's do it, then. I'm ready."

Dr. Kumar allows me to readjust my position, and then he injects me with a local anesthetic again to numb the pain. However, this time it is higher up my back. There is no question. I can feel this baby.

Shit! Even the small needle really hurts. What is that big one going to be like?

I hear Terry and Shelly talking in the background. Shelly comes over and wipes my brow with a cool towel.

"You're being very brave," she says softly.

"Thanks. I appreciate you saying that."

And I do. It helps me to brace myself for round two. Actually, this is round three, seeing as they have already tried one needle and switched to a second, bigger needle.

I can't take much more of this. Let's just get it over with as quickly as possible.

"Dr. Kumar!"

"Yes? Is the area numb, Matthew?"

"Not sure. Probably." I am talking as fast as I can. "Why don't you just go ahead and use the big needle from the start? It's worth it to not have to go in twice again."

He is quiet for a minute. He probably thinks he has a masochist on his hands. "Are you sure you want to do that?" he asks.

Whoa. What does it mean when your calm, rational doctor asks you if you're sure about something? Am I nuts? But what other options do I have? I want this over. I want my feet, legs, penis, everything, to return to what I was before. If this is what I have to do, then so be it.

"I have faith in you," I tell him.

Then I realize that sounds ridiculous, so I add, "We've shared so many intimate moments over the past couple of days. Why stop now?"

Shelly and Terry laugh. Dr. Kumar remains all business.

Hey, by the way ... how has my spine calcified? What is that all about? Am I not drinking enough milk?

"Ready?" Dr. Kumar asks, snapping me back to reality.

"As ready as I'm ever going to be."

I assume the position again with my elbows square on the table and my head resting in my hands. The pressure begins. This time it seems to be in the middle of my back. A sharp shooting sensation spreads down the left side of my body. Instantly, the pressure mounts.

I dig my nails into the side of my head.

There is some discussion behind me, muffled by the strange sensations my body is now experiencing. Shelly is visibly concerned, but stands strong in front of me.

"Matthew," she says, "I'm here. Let me know if you need anything."

"Thanks," I manage to spit out, along with some stale saliva.

The pressure is getting difficult to bear. I feel as though I am being sliced in half. Is this supposed to be happening? My entire body has become rigid and unable to turn. I am also afraid to move my head in any direction. I clench my fists.

Sweat pours out of me. The pain is excruciating. I start pulling hard on my hair, trying not to yell. But it cannot be helped.

"ARGHHHHH!"

"Do you need a break, Matthew?"

"Are we in?"

"Yes," he replies.

"Then I don't need a break."

I can feel salty sweat on my lips. My body temperature is shooting up. I look toward the floor and see my leg muscles spasming, kicking uncontrollably … but I can't feel myself kicking.

Then my arms start to shake. My head is too heavy in my hands. I lift it slightly. Slow and straight, trying to minimize spinal movements. I reach to the edge of the table and grip harder. Then I drop my head, not caring about the consequence.

"ARGHHH!" A thunderbolt of pain shoots up my neck.

"Let's stop," Dr. Kumar says.

"Are we finished?"

"No," he says. "We are in position now, and I need to collect the fluid."

Wait. He hasn't even started taking my fluid yet? Shit! What is the next course? Death?

"Keep going then," I somehow muster the courage to say. "Let's get it over with."

"Okay," Dr. Kumar responds. "I am going to start the extraction. I need to fill four separate tubes for different tests."

I steel myself again. This is like taking blood, right? It takes seconds to fill a tube with blood. This should be over in a minute, I tell myself. I roll my eyes at Shelly.

"I'm here for you, Matthew."

Now there is a strange metallic taste in my mouth. Hmm. I start lapping the roof of my mouth with my tongue. Odd. I can't explain it, but it is there. I keep lapping my mouth with my tongue, like I am chewing a sour lemon. It isn't going away. It scares me enough to mention it to Dr. Kumar.

"Doc, my mouth—"

"What is it?"

"—the inside. It kind of tastes like, umm, well, like formaldehyde."

"Formaldehyde?" He sounds perplexed. "And what does formaldehyde taste like, exactly?"

Hey, I'm not the doctor! But, weirdly, trying to answer that question does take my mind off the procedure for a bit. I pause for what seemed like forever. It is getting difficult to string together complete thoughts.

"What does it …? I don't know. Slow death?"

He pauses. "Riiiight. Well, patients do tend to experience strange taste sensations. This is totally normal. You are doing fine."

"Are we almost finished?"

"Well, unfortunately not. The spinal fluid is not coming out as fast as we would like. It is sort of a slow drip. We have not filled the first tube yet. Hang in there. You're doing fine."

My calculations are way off. Shit, shit, shit.

Shelly jumps in. "You're doing awesome, Matt. Keep it up!"

The shooting pain now moves up my body from the point of the needle insertion and spreads out over my arms and lower neck. I lean forward and arch my back.

I desperately try to generate saliva to make the awful taste in my mouth disappear. I am way past sweaty. It's like I am swimming in a pool of my own making. I feel nauseated, like I am going to vomit any second.

The room is getting hotter and hotter. And hotter.

"Argggghhhhh!!!!!!!!!!!"

Yeah, right. No pain. No pain. They meant KNOW pain. I did not know pain. Until today.

"Matt," Dr. Kumar says again, "try to hold still."

"I'm trying! I'm trying!" I hear myself yelling at him.

Shelly wipes the sweat from my brow.

"I need to take off my Johnny!" I cry. "It's so hot in here. I'm dying."

Shelly reaches around my neck and grabs the Johnny, pulling it forward. The pressure in my back continues to mount. She helps it down my arms. I grab for it with my hands, but my range of movement is limited to bending only from the elbows down. I feel like my spine has been severed from the needle down. I grab for the corner of Johnny so I can wipe my face.

"Hold still, Matthew!"

Fuck it. I can't take it anymore. I pull the Johnny off my body, ball it up, and wipe the sweat off my face. I am sitting there in just boxers with my penis hanging out the opening, choking on a plastic catheter tube. So much for being self-conscious.

"Argggghhhhh."

"You're doing great Matthew. We're almost there." He sounds almost encouraging.

Shelly puts her hand on my forehead. "Terry, get me a damp towel. He's burning up!"

I arch my back out further and scrape my elbows along the table. I clench my fists so hard I think my fingernails are breaking through the skin of my palms. And I have no fingernails because I bite them. My hands are stinging, but I keep squeezing harder and harder, trying to force the spinal fluid out of my back and into these damn tubes.

"I need a drink!" I scream.

The response isn't fast enough. Don't they know I am dehydrated and dying?

"Water, please! I need water NOW!"

Shelly pours me a cup and raises it to my lips.

I am shaking. "Shelly," I pant. "I'm so hot. I'm sooooooo sick."

"I know, Matthew, I know." She reaches her hands toward mine. "Hold my hands if you need to," she says.

I unclench my fists and grab hers, clamping down like a vice. Her face turns red.

"Is that too tight?" I gasp.

She shakes her head.

Then more pain hits. I am dying. I know it.

"You are doing great, Matthew. Just two more tubes to go," Dr. Kumar informs me.

Two more tubes? The needle has been in me forever by now. What am I? A freakin' maple tree? Spinal fluid seeping from my body like sap? Are four tubes really necessary? I am more and more nauseated and sweating a river. There is a constant pain shooting down the side of my body. My legs are locked. I am feeling deathly ill.

I look down in front of me.

"Oh, Shelly," I say. "Sorry about your hands."

She actually laughs. "You're doing great, Matt. This isn't half as hard as how I squeezed my husband's hand in the delivery room. Just keep fighting."

I close my eyes again and squeeze tighter to keep my sweaty, slippery hands from sliding out of her grasp.

"One more, Matthew," Dr. Kumar says.

One more.

Think of something different, Matt. So it doesn't hurt. Take *your mind away from what's going on.* I squeeze harder and harder. I look at my balled fists squeezing Shelly's hands. I expect to see blood oozing through the cracks in my fingers.

Somehow, Terry gets a hold of a cold, damp towel and

wipes down my face and chest. Sweat continues to pour down my brow, blurring my vision. I can still faintly see Shelly. She looks at me, then at the doctor, then back at me like there is something incredibly wrong.

God, this is crazy! It must be approaching an hour now, and I still have an epidural-sized needle stuck smack dab in the middle of my back. It is draining the life from my spine. I start to gag on my own tongue. I choke a little, turn my head away from Shelly, and spit at the wall. I can not bear the astringent taste any longer. My nausea increases, and I feel feverish and weak. I can no longer battle the shooting pain. I am paralyzed from the waist down, I can't feel nor move my legs, and every muscle in my body is tense to the point of rigor mortis.

But I am in the home stretch. No quitting now. I look past Shelly and concentrate on the rainy window and angry sky. I try to straighten my leg, but the pain snaps it back down. I lose my grip on Shelly's hands and start to collapse on my side. She does not allow that. She grabs my hands tighter and looks me in the eyes with a look that tells me she isn't going to let me go. We are in this together.

Then...

"Matthew, we are finished now."

And just like that, it is over.

I feel something pull on my back, and the pressure is instantly released. Calm surrounds me. Time seems to slow down. Shelly lets go of my hands. I slump over to my left and slide down on the mattress, coming to rest on my side. Shelly, Terry, and Dr. Kumar huddle at the foot of my bed, but I can't make out what they are saying, they are so far away from me, and there is a strange rushing noise in my ears, almost like I am listening through a sea shell.

There is movement now. Terry wheels the tray out through the curtain. Dr. Kumar sits on the chair beside my bed and writes notes on my chart. Shelly gently lifts my legs onto the bed.

The room is spinning now. I try to focus my eyes. My body is drenched in sweat, my hair completely soaked, my boxers all twisted, my penis and catheter tube exposed for everyone to see. But I just don't care. Sprawled out on the bed, staring blankly at the ceiling, I feel like an appliance that has just been unplugged.

The medical staff reassembles at the foot of my bed. My hearing is still faulty, so I start to pull myself up to see what is going on, but Terry quickly rushes to my side.

"Matthew, it is extremely important to remain lying down," she says. "I cannot stress to you how important this is."

My eyes are still not functioning. She moves too fast for my pupils to process her motion. I am seeing trails of green and yellow energy behind her.

"Okay," I reply, confused. I fall back onto the pillow.

Then it hits me. Forget the exhaustion. The effects of the spinal tap finally register. Pain and lots of it. I am not even sure where it is coming from. My hair, my skin, my limbs, my eyes, my head, my everything. It seems to radiate from every cell in my body. My entire being is sensitive to the slightest movement. Even the stale air of the room pressing against my skin is more than I can bear.

"I need drugs," I whimper. "I'm in pain."

"Can you rate the pain?" Shelly asks.

I pause, just to gather my strength to answer her question. "It's a ten," I say. "At least a ten. Shelly, please!"

Dr. Kumar is standing over me, but when I look up at him, I can barely see his face. My eyes are stinging, as if my retinas have been singed by fire.

"Well, Matthew, your brain is partially supported by your spine, and the spinal fluid is like hydraulic fluid. When we take the fluid from your spine, your brain sinks a little to the bottom of your skull. If you lie back and keep still, you will be okay. If not, you will feel a lot of pain."

Is he talking through a megaphone? His voice is amplified like he is screaming at me. Then it drops down to a low murmur.

I suck in some air. Shit! It is like I have just inhaled next to an open fire.

"How'd we do?" I moan.

Dr. Kumar smiles and raises four tubes for me to see. It takes a moment for me to train my vision on these tiny tubes. They resemble the kind used to collect blood. Each is filled about a quarter of the way up. I can't believe I sweated and groaned for such a miserly amount of fluid. Three tubes have clear fluid, but one tube has a red tint. Is that my blood mixed in it?

It doesn't matter now. Not with my entire body in a pain seizure.

"Drugs. Morphine! Please!" I plead.

My head is throbbing now. At first it feels like someone has my brain in their hands and is rubbing it against a large rock. But with this new pulsating sensation, it feels like, along with the scraping, someone else is also beating it with a hammer.

Just then Jocelyn walks into the room. For some reason, the sight of her makes me lose the last of my inhibitions.

"Help me!" I scream. "This pain is too much. PLEASE HURRY!"

She is by my side, holding my head. She looks panicked.

"Joci, please," I beg her. "You've got to help me. I need drugs. I need drugs now!"

I am panting. I need air. But the air that I am breathing feels like it is full of tiny pieces of metal. As I suck it in, I feel it ripping the lining of my lungs.

"Aaaaarrrggghhhh!" I try to push the poisonous air

out.

Shelly runs back into the room. "They have to hand-carry your prescription from another floor because it's a narcotic," she says, out of breath. "We don't have it on this floor."

"Oh, fuck ... oh, fuck ... oh, fuck." I don't want to hear about the fucking bureaucracy. "Just get me something! Anything! NOW!"

Jocelyn is somehow holding my hand. "Be strong, baby, I'm here." She sits down next to me and dabs my forehead with a damp towel. It hurts. I don't want anyone touching me. Not even her.

Shelly appears next to my bed. "Drugs—Shelly. Please, now!"

"Matt, I've been on the phone. They're rushing the prescription up. It'll be here soon."

I am out of breath. Consumed with fear and pain and nausea.

Someone runs into the room. All I see are blue scrubs. "Nurse!"

Someone is carrying a clear liquid in a clear plastic bag. She hangs it on the IV pole and plugs it into my tube.

"You'll be fine," she says calmly. "It will kick in any second."

I lie flat, helpless, paralyzed with fear. My sheets are damp and twisted around me from my struggle. I watch the medicine flow down the tube and into my arm.

I feel a sharp pain over my forehead, like I've been struck by a lightning bolt. It splits my skull in half. The rain running down the window sounds like nails on a chalkboard. The room is a spinning, a blurry mix of shadows and colors. I have never experienced such searing pain.

Then it happens. The drug starts to seep into my soul.

I am transported to a quiet place, somewhere void of lights and sound. The torture is over. For now.

Chapter Seventeen - Thursday, May 26

The rain continues its incessant pounding against my window, masked by the black of night. A nurse has just been in to take my vital signs, draw blood, refresh my pain medicine and re-tape my IV.

The glow from the TV illuminates the room like a low hanging full moon. I'm trying to watch the TV, but I'm having trouble focusing my eyes. Sound, too, is muffled and distant, like I have ear plugs in. It's an entirely different dimension of being. Nothing seems real anymore.

I wipe my left hand, the one without the IV in it, over my face, clearing the sleep out of my eyes. The skin of my face feels fat, flush, warm, and my five o'clock shadow is fast turning into a prickly beard. My mouth is dry. I can't wash the metallic taste out.

I raise my right hand in front of my eyes, but I don't have the strength to keep it steady. Swirling, flickering lights trail behind my fingers as I try to look more closely at the damn IV. Its rhythmic beat is playing over and over in my head.

The IV meter beeps.

Then hisses.

Then splashes.

One drop.

One tiny droplet of medicine at a time drops out of the bag to swim down through the clear plastic tube and eventually enter my body. The repetitive nature of the process, along with the beat of the machine, has a hypnotic effect on me.

My eyes are dry. My eyelids are heavy. I'm barely hanging on, but I'm still fixated on the three IV bags above my head. What's even in there? I need to ask more questions.

Beep

Hiss
Splash
Drop

~~~

My cell phone is ringing. What time is it? The Arizona
sun is already pelting our bedroom window but it is still too
early to get up. Especially since it's Memorial Day- no classes
or work today. The incessant pinging of the cell phone ring
tone is agonizing my hung over brain. I am in the bedroom
lying next to Jocelyn and the phone is ringing somewhere out
in the kitchen. After a moment, the ringing stops and I turn
back over to go to sleep.

Then it starts again. I look at the clock on Jocelyn's side
of the bed. It is only 6:30. I close my eyes and let the cell
phone go to voicemail again.

For a third time the cell phone starts ringing and I
know someone needs to talk to me.

I instantly think that something is wrong. I propel
myself out of bed and head to the kitchen.

I grab the phone off the counter and see that I have
three missed calls from my Dad. He never calls more than
once. My first thought is of my Grandmother. She is in her
late eighties and battling an onset of dementia. Maybe this is
a phone call that I don't want to return.

I carefully dial the number and take a deep breath.

The phone rings.

"Hello"

"Hi Dad, it's 6:30 in the morning out here." I whisper,
"What's going on?"

"Sorry, Matt. I wasn't thinking about the time. Hey,
are you sitting down?"

"No why?"

"I have to tell you something."

"Hold on." I pick up my jeans off the floor from the night before, put them on and walk out onto our back patio.

"Ok, we can talk now Dad. What's up?"

"Something happened to Zack." He says somberly.

"What do you mean?" My heart leaps to my throat.

"He got out of the house and wandered up to the road. A little old lady was coming over the hill and ah um, he wasn't able to get out of the way."

"NO!" I gasp.

"Matt, it isn't what you think. She barely tapped him. He was old and his hips were failing. She hit him going like ten miles per hour and then he walked down the bottom of the driveway, laid down and closed his eyes. He was in peace. We were going to have to put him down. This is a blessing in a way."

"But I didn't get to say goodbye."

"You two had a good life together. By the time you left for college, his best years were behind him. German Shepherds are such great dogs, but they break down so quickly."

"You think it was because I left? I mean he didn't even get to meet Jocelyn."

"This would've happened whether you were here or not. While you were here, you guys had a great time together."

"Ok, thanks Dad. I just wish I could've said goodbye."

I hang up the phone and collapse on the patio chair. I start crying uncontrollably feeling that I have betrayed my dog by not saying goodbye. I fire up cigarette.

Staring up at the blue sky, I cry aloud between puffs, "Damnit Zack...I needed you to hold on until summer so you could meet Jocelyn...I'm sorry I wasn't there...You were always there for me...I'm gonna miss you buddy!" Then squinting at the sunlight, I whisper, "Goodbye my puppy."

~~~

"Matt?"

I bury my head under the pillow.

"Matt?"

A soft hand is on my shoulder.

"Matt, wake up," Jocelyn shakes me gently.

I squint out of my troubled dream.

"What? What is it?" I say groggily.

"Gerard's on the phone."

"Gerard?" I am confused. Where am I?

"Your boss."

Oh. I gather myself together. My eyes roll around the room, my head still floating from narcotics. Oh, yeah, I'm in the hospital. I take the phone from Jocelyn. "Hello?" I say, in as macho a voice as I can muster.

"Matt?" a cheerful, familiar voice responds.

"Yes?"

"This is Gerard."

"Gerard! Hi, how are you?"

"I'm fine."

I can feel him smiling over the telephone line.

"The big question is, how are you doing?"

Jocelyn tries to get my attention. She is waving at me and pointing at a bouquet of flowers on the window sill. Aaaah, those must be from the company.

I raise my index finger and gesture that I will express thanks in a minute. "Well, Gerard, I've been better. I've been through a lot the past couple of days."

"Sorry to hear that."

"They've put me through a battery of tests including CAT scans, MRIs, and x-rays. And, most recently, a spinal tap."

"Wow. You have been through a lot. You poor guy. How ya feeling?"

"The spinal tap just happened yesterday, so I'm resting now. I don't feel any different yet, but I've got so much pain medication in me that I can't feel anything. I'm just trying to rest up and return to work as soon as possible. Hopefully by next Monday."

"Matt, don't worry about work right now," he says. "You have to concentrate on getting better. Your position will be here waiting for you when you're able to return. We all want to see you, but we want you to come back healthy."

"Really? Hey, that's great, Gerard. That means a lot to me. It really does. Oh, and thank you for the flowers. They're beautiful."

"No problem." He laughs. "It's the least we could do. We're pulling for you over here, big guy. We miss having you around the office."

I feel a little choked up. It is probably the narcotics. "That means a lot to me," I say. "I just wish that I could've been there to help with the big move. How's the new office space, by the way?"

"The new place is great. I can't wait to show it to you. The move went smoothly. We have you all set up in a cubicle by a window. The only thing missing is you."

"Thank you, Gerard. I really appreciate talking to you today and I hope I'll see you soon."

"Take care, Matt. I hope everything works out okay. Bye now."

"Bye, Gerard. Thanks again."

I hang up the phone and smile at Jocelyn. "Well, at least I still have a job. I didn't think anyone would want to keep me around now that I am damaged goods," I say, only half joking.

The truth is that the whole time I have been in the hospital I have been worried that everyone would turn their backs on me — work, family, friends, even Jocelyn. When I look at my wife, I see a woman who is much too young to care for a sick husband for the rest of her life. She can easily find another man who is healthy. I don't want to be a burden. Not to her. Not to anybody.

Jocelyn looks at me with intense eyes, leans over, and kisses me gently on the forehead. "Well," she says with a wink, "you're stuck with me, no matter what. And don't you ever forget it!" She winks again.

I smile.

Chapter Eighteen - Physical Therapy Assessment

I don't know what happened to lunch. I must have dozed off. As I rub my eyes, a woman about my age with blonde hair, a bright smile and dark blue scrubs is coming through the door.

"Hi. My name is Kristen. I will be your physical therapist."

"Hi Kristen," I say.

I am enjoying the pain medicine and beginning to feel like the host of a talk show. Lying in bed is like sitting at the host's desk with different people wandering into the room to be interviewed.

"So," I say, "am I going to get physical therapy now?"

"That's what they tell me." She smiles again.

"Really? What does that entail?"

"Nothing too strenuous," she replies. "I've just got to get you up and walking."

"Um," I say, "have you cleared this with the nurses?"

"Yes. This is standard procedure." She glances at her clipboard.

I am skeptical. "You do know that I had a spinal tap yesterday?"

I can see Jocelyn inching forward with a look of concern on her face.

Kristen consults her clipboard again. "Yes. It says that right here. But they want you to do some walking."

Jocelyn can't contain herself any longer. "But Shelly told him he wasn't to move at all. He's supposed to lie on his back so he doesn't get the bad headaches from the spinal tap."

"Shelly said that, huh?" Kristen sounds puzzled. "It

says here that they want to start you walking. If you don't think you can do it, though, I can always come back tomorrow."

I am starting to put two and two together. Not that I have figured out anything especially complex, but it is becoming apparent to me that I will not be leaving this hospital until I can show them that I can walk again. My new friend, Kristen, is going to be crucial in getting my ticket home.

But Jocelyn is concerned. "He's had a really tough twenty four hours," she explains. "I don't know if he should walk today."

I interrupt her. "How far do I have to walk?"

"Just down the hall and back," Kristen replies.

I look at Jocelyn, pleading with her, really. Then I turn back to Kristen. "So, Kristen, I have to show everyone I can walk before they'll let me out of here?"

She looks down at the clipboard again. "That's what it says."

"Well, I guess today is as good a day as any to try walking again." I start to get out of bed.

Kristen unplugs the IV from the wall and rolls it forward. The IV monitor starts to beep. She then presses a button on the monitor and the beeping stops. The IV medicine, however, continues to drip. If I am going to try to walk, I am going to need all the help I can get.

She puts her free arm inside my arm. I place my left hand down on the bed and push myself up. I freeze for a minute as the blood rushes from my brain and black dots speckle my vision. Am I going to black out?

I gather myself, the haze lifts, and the dots clear. I reach down and pick up my catheter bag and hold it firmly on my left side.

"Do you need a cane?"

"No. I'm good. I think." My macho Italian pride

returns along with the blood to my brain.

I free myself from Kristen's hands and attempt to do the penguin walk out the door. Penguin walking is difficult to do, however, while holding a bag of urine. I notice my roommate is awake. He waves to me.

"What's up, dude?" I ask.

"Nothing much, man," he responds. "Good luck!"

"Thanks."

As I stumble toward the wall, Kristen reaches out to grab me and steady me on course. She puts her left arm around the small of my back and forces my right arm up over her shoulder. She rolls the IV pole with her right hand.

She is good at this.

"You do realize," I say, "that if I lose my balance and fall, I may crush you?"

"You'll do fine," she assures me. "Let's take a right out the door and go down the hall."

We continue at a slow pace. I have been immobile for so long that I am having a hard time remembering how to walk, so my steps are slow and unsteady. Kristen is holding me tighter as we make our way down the corridor.

"You know, despite what it seems, I really can walk."

"I know you can."

"It is just that I have had a very traumatic past few days and this bag of urine isn't really instilling any confidence in me."

She giggles a little but tries to maintain her composure. My guess is that most people who need to learn how to walk again generally take it more seriously than me.

We pass the nurses' station, where Terry and Shelly are sitting. I smile as I stroll by and said, "Hey, I know you two!"

"A little happier, are we?" Shelly asks.

"A little bit. I think I'd be happier if I wasn't lugging around a bag of pee."

We continue on at a snail's pace.

"Do you think you can make it to the end of the hall?" Kristen asks.

"Wow." I take a look. "That's pretty far away. My head is starting to hurt. I think I've had enough fun for today."

"Come on," she insists. "You're doing a great job. Let's go the distance!" She is really excited.

"Great job?" I say sarcastically. "I don't know if I'd go that far."

My head is starting to pound. It is like someone has put a garbage can over it and is pounding it randomly. My vision is blurring, too, and saliva starts to ooze in my mouth. I swallow hard. *Fight through it.*

Kristen apparently notices. "Do you really want to turn around?" she asks.

"I'm on some kind of pain med because my spinal fluid was drained," I say. "My back hurts and my head is throbbing. I know I can walk. Just not right now."

The walk is not going well now. Even with her holding me, I am stumbling into the wall. I have no sense of balance, and the pee bag in my hand totally eliminates my equilibrium. I need to lie down. I can't make it any farther.

But she looks at me with determination.

I am not going to let her down. I need a good report. "You know what?" I say. "Let's finish the hallway. My bed will still be there when I get back."

"You sure?"

"Not really. But if that's what you want me to do, I will do it."

We continue down the hall. Slow, uneven step after slow, uneven step.

Then, suddenly, toward the end of the hall, a pain as fast and furious as lightning strikes through my skull. This must be the headache they have been forecasting. It is like nothing I have ever experienced before. You can't call this a headache. This comes deep from the bowels of hell. It is so violent and intense that I can't focus on anything.

My eyes blur. I try to speak. Drool runs down my chin. I begin to wobble back and forth. My left knee collapses and Kristen loses her grip on my arm. She has been supporting me, and without her help, I tumble to the floor, dropping the bag of pee on my way down.

"OH, MY GOD! Help! Help!" she yells.

I don't have the strength to do or say anything, but as Shelly and Terry come running, I try to pull myself together. I am lying in the middle of a hallway on my back in a hospital gown with a bag of pee beside me. But none of this matters. My head is being electrocuted.

The girls are talking up above me. Their conversation is like white noise in my fried brain. I lie still, frozen by the fireworks in my head. After what seems like forever, little by little, my senses start creeping back. The voltage drops. The saliva slows, and my eyes clear. The grand finale of the fireworks display in my brain is over.

I reach up with one hand. "I think that's enough for today," I joke. "Here. Help me up?"

"No. You stay right there. We've called for a wheelchair."

I lie and wait for the wheelchair to arrive. For the first time in this process, I give in. I can't help it. The wheelchair. The possible MS. Memories of my aunt Loretta. It's all too overwhelming and real.

Two male orderlies arrive, faster than I expect, and stand on either side of me. They bend down, reach under my shoulders, and pull me to my feet.

"Sit back, Matthew," Shelly's familiar voice is behind me.

I sit back onto the firm leather seat of the wheelchair. One of the orderlies picks my legs up, one at a time, and sets my feet on the metal footrest.

We are off. We make it back to Emerson 484.

Then Jocelyn sees me in the wheelchair. "Oh, my God! What happened?" She rushes to my side.

"It's nothing, baby," I smile weakly. "I just fell, I'm fine."

They push me past my roommate, who has returned to his snoring state, and up to my bed. Then the orderlies pull me out of the chair and lay me on the bed. I lie back and rest my head on the pillow.

Shelly rushes to my side with two pills and a cup of water.

"Thank you," I say, and swallow the pills.

Kristen is standing next to Jocelyn at the foot of my bed.

"How'd he do?" Jocelyn asks her, not taking her eyes off of me.

"He did okay," Kristen says. "But I think we might want to wait a day or two before we try again."

"I'll be fine. I can do it tomorrow," I counter, ignoring the doubt that the atom bomb headache has drilled into my psyche.

Kristen smiles at me. "Well, I like your spirit. I'll come by tomorrow, and if you're ready, we'll try it again. If not, no big whoop. We'll wait till the next day."

I look at her hard. "I'll be ready to walk tomorrow."

"Okay. Well, you take care and I'll see you tomorrow."

The fall and wheelchair transport have scared me more than a little bit. I have to be able to walk again. No matter what the cost. I refuse to let whatever is happening to me get the best of me! I'm gonna walk all right. Right on outta here. And get back to living my life.

Chapter Nineteen - Friday, May 27

"Shelly?" It is morning. Shelly is fussing with my IV. "Have you talked to the doctors?"

She just smiles.

"No, really," I persist. "Am I going home this morning? I have some feeling back. See? Pinch me."

I pull the sheet back and expose my thigh. Then I playfully pinch myself.

She giggles. "Well, good, Matt. I'm glad you're starting to feel better." She turns away, but keeps fiddling with the IV. "Matt ... I ... uh ... I ... don't think you're going home today."

My mood shifts. She has caught me off-guard.

"Umm ... wait.... Why?"

"Well," she pauses, "a couple of things. You need to demonstrate that you can walk and pee on your own. After yesterday, Kristen is going to recommend that you stay here at least another day. We also need to remove the catheter so you can demonstrate that you can pee on your own."

I blink my eyes. "Demonstrate??"

"Well, yeah ... there's a pitcher we're going to ask you to fill."

"An entire pitcher?"

"Yes," she answers matter-of-factly. Then she remembers something. "Actually," she says, "I can see if Dr. Titleman will authorize removing the catheter. I'll go do that now."

That's when Jocelyn walks in. The entire room seems to brighten.

"Good morning, Shelly. How is Mr. Grumpy this morning?"

"He wants to go home," Shelly says. "Surprisingly."

They talk like I am not even in the room. I look up at the TV and check the weather forecast.

Looks like the rain has finally run its course. Spring might have finally sprung—just in time for summer!

"Hey, look!" I point up at the TV, stopping Jocelyn and Shelly mid-conversation. "The storm is lifting. It's going to be a perfect day." I pause meaningfully. "A perfect day for me to go home, that is."

Shelly giggles again. "Well, you know what you have to do, Mister. Like I said, the consensus around here is that you're staying another day. You'll have to pull off a miracle for that to happen."

I look over at Jocelyn. Then back at Shelly. "I'm in the business of pulling off miracles, Shelly. I'm leaving today!"

"Well, I'm pulling for you. In the meantime, I'll send Dr. Titleman in to see you shortly and he can explain everything."

Shelly walks out.

Jocelyn comes over and kisses me on the forehead, and then she sits at my bedside and rests her hand in mine. "So, how is my baby feeling today?"

"I'm fine," I grumble. "I just want to go home."

"Did you get any feeling back in your legs?" she asks.

"I don't know. Maybe. Pinch me."

She lifts my blanket and pinches me playfully.

"OUCH!"

She jumps three feet in the air. "Oh, my God!" she cries. "I'm sorry, baby!"

The look on her face is priceless.

"I'm kidding!" I laugh. "But actually I did feel it a little. Slowly but surely, everything seems to be coming back to life."

As if on cue, Dr. Titleman walks in the room. "Good morning, Matthew," he says stiffly.

"Good morning, Dr. Titleman," I respond in like

fashion.

"So, you think you are ready to go home today?" he asks as he flips through my chart.

"Do I have any more tests?"

"No." He responds matter-of-factly.

"How about medicine? Am I finished with that?"

"For the most part. Yes. Although you are going to be switched to an oral steroid regimen."

I pause. "So ... no more IV medicine. Correct?"

"Yes, that is correct." He is addressing the clipboard, not looking at me.

"Then I would like to go home today."

He ignores me and continues flipping through the chart. Then, "Do you have any feeling back in your lower half?"

"My thighs have some sensation," I say, "and my lower legs and feet, too. I'm sure I'll know if I have sensations back in my genitals when the catheter is removed."

He puts my chart down and looks into my eyes with a stern seriousness. "Okay, there are going to be a couple of things you have to do before I release you. One, I want to remove the catheter and have you produce one liter of urine on your own. Two, I want you to work with the physical therapist again to prove that you are safe on your feet. I cannot release you if you cannot go to the bathroom on your own or if you continue to be a fall risk."

A challenge, huh? Does he doubt my steely resolve?

"Well, I'm ready for those tests," I say curtly. "So the sooner we begin, the sooner I can go."

"Okay then," he picks up the chart again, closes it, and finally acknowledges me. "I will send Shelly in to remove the catheter and to give you your sample bottle to urinate in. The physical therapist will be making her rounds in the afternoon, so you will probably be here at least until three or four o'clock."

I nod. "Thank you, Dr. Titleman. I guarantee you that I will pass these tests, so whenever you want to get started, I'm ready."

He tucks the clipboard under his arm, turns, and walks out.

There is no way I am going to spend another night in this room. But what scares me the most right now isn't the walking; I am more worried about having to produce so much pee.

But I have an idea. Oh, yes. That urine jug is no match for Matt Cavallo at full throttle.

"Jocelyn, would you mind handing me the phone and getting me a glass of water, please?"

She looks at me curiously, but hands me the phone and then goes to ask the nurse for some spring water. I dial and wait for an answer on the other end. "Hi, Mom," I say.

"How's my boy?"

"I'm fine. Are you planning on coming over here this morning, or are you working?"

"I'm supposed to be at work around two, but I was planning on coming over this morning. Why?"

"Well, here is what I need you to do. Can you swing by Dunkin' Donuts and get me a large hot coffee and a large iced coffee, both with cream and sugar?"

"Why do you want that much coffee? I don't think you should be drinking that much."

"Don't worry about it now, Ma. It's doctor's orders."

"Really? Okay. I'm on my way."

Twenty minutes or so pass. I drink all the water in the small gray pitcher that comes with the morning meal. Then I proceed to drink the small bottle of cranberry juice. I can't wait until my Mom gets here with the coffee.

Shelly enters the room, carrying a plastic pitcher with measuring cup lines on it. She smiles at me. I can't believe it. It looks like the size of a garbage pail.

"I have to fill that up?" I squeak.

She nods.

I look at the pitcher again and realize it would probably take a good six to twelve beers to fill that thing within a reasonable amount of time. Seeing as the beers are not an option, I am banking on the coffee. Coffee makes me pee, but it also has an unwanted side effect: nicotine fits.

"Are you ready?" she asks.

"Ready for what?"

"I'm going to take your catheter out."

"What about my IV? Can you take that out, too?" She shakes her head. "Sorry. We can't do that until your release is authorized."

"I don't know if I want to see this," Jocelyn says from her chair at the foot of the bed.

Shelly smiles at her. "It'll only take a second. You can wait in the hallway, and I'll come get you when I'm finished."

"Okay." Sounding relieved, she stands up and quickly leaves the room as Shelly walks over to my bed and lifts up my Johnny.

I flinch a little as she begins.

"Just relax," she says. She is all business now as she lifts my Johnny higher and starts fiddling around with the line that went from me to the urine bag.

I can't see what she is doing down there with the bunched up Johnny in the way, but I have a feeling this is going to hurt a bit. I am hoping I will feel something. Well, maybe not screeching pain. But it would be nice to feel something.

"Shelly," I ask. "Are you going to give me any warning?"

She is focused on her work. "I just have to get the catheter ready to remove it."

"I'm ready now," she says. "Are you?"

I grip the side of the bed. "Ready as I'll ever be!"

"Okay. Brace yourself."

She rustles the sheets a bit, and then starts to pull the tube out of my penis.

I wince a little and turn my head. It is fine for a second, but then a searing pain scorches inside me. I blanch.

"Are you okay?" she asks.

"IT BURNS!"

"Really?" She laughs. "You should be happy."

I look down at my penis and see its mouth open wide as the tube comes sliding out. It is unnatural to see it stretched out like that. The burning sensation is strong.

"Happy?" I groan. "Why?"

"Because you have your feeling back."

Huh?

Wow.

She is right.

She is right!

I pump my fist in triumph, "Yes!"

The catheter tube is completely out of me. I cover myself up and get situated as Shelly puts the bag and tube in a plastic container and begins to clean up.

"That's great, Matt!" she says.

"Fantastic!" I cry out.

She shoots me a look like I am getting a little carried away. "Now," she says, "do you think you can pee for me?"

"I don't know," I mumble as I look down and feel around my bladder. "No, not yet."

She looks disappointed.

"It will happen soon," I say convincingly.

With a little help from my friends at Dunkin' Donuts, that is.

Chapter Twenty - Hospital Discharge

It is almost lunchtime, and the pee container is nearly half full. My plan is working brilliantly.

Kristen bounces in the room. It looks like she has put yesterday's failure behind her.

"Are you ready, Matthew?"

"Sure!" I shout out, equaling her enthusiasm. "What are we going to do today?"

She doesn't realize that I am super-charged on two super-sized coffees. If she asks me to fly, I probably will sprout wings and leap into the air.

"Let's try what we did yesterday," she says. "I brought you a cane this time. Do you think you can make it?"

I look at her. "If I start walking with this thing does that mean you classify me as walking? And I can check the box to get out of this place?"

She nods.

"Hey, no problem then. You're the boss. Let's go." I slip over the side of the bed and stand up, though precariously.

She gives me a wary look. "Have you walked with a cane before?"

I think for a second. "Uh, no."

"Well, this is how you do it. Hold the cane in your right hand and put it down with your left foot."

She demonstrates the cane walk. I concentrate on her demonstration.

"Okay," I say. "Looks easy enough."

She hands me the cane, and I start hobbling out of the room with it, but I keep putting it down with the right foot. I look back at her. "Sorry, I just can't figure this out. I'm left handed."

She smiles. "Okay, then try putting the cane in your left hand and coming down on your right foot."

It feels goofy at first, but then I hit my stride. And when I realize I am actually walking fairly well with the cane, it charges me up even more. All of a sudden, I have superhuman strength pumping through me. It is amazing what I am feeling, being this close to getting out of this hospital.

When I am at the door of my room, I look back at Kristen and smile. I ditch the cane, leaning it against the wall, stand up straight, and glide out into the hall.

Stride after sure stride.

I make a sharp right and walk at a steady pace down the hallway. I have no idea where this strength and ability to walk are coming from.

Oh, yeah. The coffee.

"Wow, this is unbelievable!" Kristen exclaims from two feet behind me. She still isn't taking any chances.

I wave as I pass the nurses' station. They look up in astonishment. I am almost running.

"Wow, look at you!" says Shelly

"I didn't know you could do that!" Terry exclaims.

"You tell Dr. Titleman I am good to go!"

We make it to the end of the hall in seconds. At that point, I am walking so fast Kristen can't keep up. I turn around and head back. Even faster now, full leg extension, like a speed walker. I high-five Shelly and Terry as I pass the nurses' station again.

Kristen looks amazed. "You are doing incredibly well, Matthew. I can't believe you are the same person I saw yesterday."

We are back at my door. "Where to next?" I ask her.

"Past your room there's a stairwell," she says. "Do you think you might try a couple of steps?"

Honey, at this point I will try to climb Mount Everest.

"Sure," I reply, confidently.

I walk over, push open the door, and look down at the steps. They are fairly wide and evenly spaced. This is going to be no problem.

I put my hand on the rail and put my right foot down on the first step.

Uh oh.

I look down to see if my foot landed safely. I put my left foot down on the next step. I can't feel it either.

"Kristen...."

"Yes"

"I just don't think I can do steps yet." I say, not wanting to give it all away.

"That's okay, Matthew. You did a great job. Let's get you back to the room."

She helps me up off the steps and I proceed to walk back to my room unassisted. My roommate looks shocked as I walk past him.

Mom is still here, sitting in a chair and reading a magazine. She looks up as I come in. "How did he do?" she asks.

Kristen is aglow. "He was amazing. I don't think I have ever seen a one-day turnaround like Matthew just had. I mean, yesterday he couldn't even balance himself, and today he is walking perfectly fine."

"So what do we do now?" Jocelyn asks.

"Initially, I was going to report that Matthew should not be discharged because of the fall risk. Now I'm going to have to change my report."

"Really?" Mom is astounded.

"Definitely. I was going to give him this cane to take home, but I'm not sure he needs it." She pauses to reconsider. "Actually," she says. "I should give it to him in case this happens again."

A chill goes up my spine. In case this happens again?

Kristen continues. "I am absolutely amazed at how well he did out there. That being said," she says, looking at me, "I want you to be careful. You still had difficulty judging the steps. I think it is important to limit your motion as much as possible. I would not recommend doing any activities that would require you to walk for an extended period of time or that require you to go up and down steps."

I laugh. "Believe me, I'm not going anywhere for awhile. So, you are going to tell Dr. Titleman that I can go home?" I cannot lose sight of my mission.

She smiles again. "Yes. I no longer view you as a fall risk. I can even take that orange sticker off of your door now."

What? That orange sticker is for me? I guess that mystery is finally solved. I am so relieved to be going home.

"Thanks, Kristen," I gush. "Thanks for everything. I promise I'll work on my pimp strut with the cane!"

After she walks out of the room, I slump back on my pillows and close my eyes. For this brief moment, everything seems okay again. Maybe this is the beginning of the end of this crazy thing I am going through. Maybe I can start my life again. Maybe ....

Then I look down at my pitcher of urine, still waiting on the table, and I know the battle is only half over.

~~~

The afternoon moves slowly. I sit up in my bed and take big gulps of more iced coffee, praying for nature to take its course. I count off the seconds, the minutes, then the hours, monitoring the swelling of my bladder. Finally, it is time. I feel a sharp pain in my side like I have been holding back for a long time.

"I have to go to the bathroom," I announce to the room.

"Do you need help?" Jocelyn answers.

I am still pumped from my session with Kristen, so I

wave her off. "Nah, I think I can do it."

I pull the sheets back, swing my legs over the side, and leverage myself out of bed. I proceed to the bathroom in good form. My confidence is evident.

"Look at you!" my roommate remarks, as I pass his open curtain.

"You're not the only one going home today!" I throw back.

"Good luck."

I walk into the bathroom, pulling the IV pole in with me, close the door, get undressed, and stare at myself in the mirror, naked with limp penis in hand. Sure, I need a shower and a shave, but I don't look sick anymore.

I put my penis inside the pitcher and hold the pitcher with my left hand. I place my right hand on the mirror and lean toward forward. My bladder releases. I feel a steady stream of pee travel through it into the tube. "Feel" is the operative word.

I sigh. It is good to feel again. At least, down there.

Then it happens.

It is as if the life escapes my body in a split second. My adrenaline level drops. My vision starts to blur. And a sledge hammer starts pounding in my brain.

I need to lie down.

Immediately.

Too late! The fireworks start again. I stumble out of the bathroom, clutching the IV pole. I don't have the strength to carry the urine pitcher.

"You don't look so good," my roommate says.

Glaciers are scraping against each other in my brain. It is an earthquake. I shuffle forward, trying to reach the sanctuary of my bed.

I can barely see. Shadows are dancing in front of my vision. I think they are trying to speak to me, but can't discern their words.

I feel arms being wrapped through my armpits. My will caves, and I feel myself being dragged. Then dropped.

Cool fresh sheets against my face.

Muffled voices and shadows buzzing about in the background.

I have been short-circuited. Completely wiped out. I need to recharge my batteries and get this headache to go away. Quick. I lie as still as can be, almost rigid. The fireworks start to play out. I keep my eyes closed tight. The muffled voices become clearer. A foreign voice comes through.

"Lunch for Mr. Cavallo."

"Put it on the table, please." Jocelyn directs.

I feel a hand on my shoulder, rubbing me gently.

I try to calm myself down. *This storm will pass, Matt.*

~~~

My eyes shoot open.

The pee pangs are brutal.

I must have passed out. Wha … what time is it? Did I miss discharge?

My abdomen is going to burst.

I can't hold back one more minute. My bladder is going to explode.

Shelly walks in to check on me. I hear her talking to my Mom and Jocelyn.

But how can I make my way to the bathroom and not suffer these excruciating headaches?

I spring up from the bed like a shot.

The crowd at the end of my bed looks as if they've seen a ghost. I grab the pitcher and turn my back to them. "Excuse me, ladies." I throw my Johnny aside and stand in my boxers in front of Jocelyn, Mom, and Shelly.

Jocelyn cries out in embarrassment. "Matt, what are

you doing?"

"I gotta go!"

A glorious stream of pee begins to rush out of me and into the pitcher. It keeps going and going and going. Second after second after second. As the pressure in my bladder diminishes, even I begin to see how absurd this scene is. I don't know whether to laugh or cry. Or blush. But as I finish, I look down. I have hit the "full" line and then some.

"I did it!" I yell triumphantly.

I turn around and raise the pitcher. "Shelly, I believe this belongs to you."

She smiles at me and takes the pitcher.

I slip back into bed, hoping I have evaded the storms in my head this time. As I lie back on the pillow, I watch Shelly walk over to the bathroom. She keeps the door open, so I can hear her pouring the pitcher into the toilet. Strange. After all that work I did, I didn't think it was just going to be poured down the toilet. I feel let down. Almost.

Shelly is back, making notes on my chart. She looks up at me and smiles. "Well, you did it. I'm going to let Dr. Titleman know. Then I think you'll be going home."

"YESSS!"

I pump my fist in excitement, but I can see that Mom and Jocelyn are concerned that I am getting too excited, so I lie back down. They are right. The last thing I need is another storm surge in my head.

Shelly returns a minute later. I can't contain myself.

"You have to take my vitals?" I ask.

"No. I'm here to take out your IV."

"YES."

I pump my fist again. I know that I have climbed the mountain. I look at Mom and Jocelyn victoriously.

Shelly begins to unwrap the layers and layers of tape that have accumulated on my wrist and arm from the adjustments various nurses have made over the past couple of days. The tape stings as it comes off, but I don't mind that in the least. Then she starts to manipulate the needle out of my wrist. It is where my wrist and the base of my thumb meet. She pulls the needle out slowly, then quickly wipes the area with rubbing alcohol and applies a Band-Aid.

I rotate my wrist a bit and work the lingering pain of the needle out of my arm. I am unable to control my smile. I know this means I will be going home shortly.

"Jocelyn," I say, "you want to throw me my clothes? I want to get changed."

She tosses me the little plastic grocery bag that holds the clothes I entered the hospital in. Sure, they have been worn and my underwear is half-past ripe, but the feeling of putting on real clothes and being out of the Johnny is more rewarding than anything I can think of. After I am dressed, I return to the bed and lie back down. I am still trying to remain conscious of the spinal tap and the necessity of keeping my head still.

Dr. Titleman walks into the room just then. Instead of walking straight to my bed, he steps inside my roommate's curtain first. I listen and squirm as he releases my roommate. My roommate walks around the curtain divider and extends his calloused hand to me. "Good luck, man" he says as he shakes my hand.

"Hey, you, too, brother." I say. Then he is gone.

Then it hits me. "Hey! What happened to Dr. Titleman? He is supposed to release me, too."

"I'm sure he'll be back to let you go soon," Mom tries to reassure me.

I am too close to the end. I can't take the anticipation. All the coffee I've had to drink is making the nicotine urge insurmountable.

I reach for my blankets. "I have to go find him," I say. "Right now!"

"No!" Mom says. "You just lie there and relax. A

minute or two won't make a difference in the long run."

I shoot Jocelyn a stare. Hoping that she will realize the urgency of getting me out of here. I am about to spiral out of control and into a nicotine fit. Actually, this is more like a nicotine rage.

My skin starts to crawl.

My chest starts to tighten.

I want to scream.

My truck. I know I need to get to my truck. There are four stale cigarettes under my car seat.

"You know," Mom says, "I think I am going to come over and help Jocelyn get you settled."

"You don't need to do that, Ma." I bark. "We're going to be okay. Plus, I know you have to get over to work."

"They don't mind if I'm a little late. They know you're here and that I want to help you."

"Well, you really won't be missing anything too exciting over at my house. I am just going to go inside and go to bed."

"I know. But I want to be there."

I ignore her pleading tone. "It's been a long week. Why don't you just stop by after dinner so I can get settled first?"

I don't want to have this battle. I want to go home with Jocelyn and have a cigarette. I know my Mom won't approve, and today is not the day to listen to her lecture me about not smoking. Why won't she just listen to me?

"But I want to help you," she repeats. "Why won't you let me help you?" Her voice is getting louder and more defensive.

I can't believe this. Is she really going to argue with me over this? What is the big deal?

I try to reason with her. "It's not that I don't want you to help me. I would just prefer to go home with Jocelyn, and then you can come and see me later."

I am getting exasperated by this conversation. Nicotine, nicotine, I need some smokes. Where the hell is Dr. Titleman?

Mom is relentless. She is not giving up. "I just don't understand why I can't come now." Her voice is also getting louder.

I can't take it anymore. "Okay, Ma." I pause and take a breath. "Here's the deal, and you're not going to like it. I don't mind you coming over, but when I get home, one of the first things I am going to do is have a cigarette. I know you don't like me smoking, but I have a lot of things on my mind right now and I am going to smoke."

The room stops. My Mom's face contorts.

I've seen this look before. Her eyes and facial features change drastically. And so begins the tirade.

"You think that I don't know about your filthy, disgusting habit!" She is already screaming. "Well, I do! I know you're a smoker! I know you try to hide it from me and everyone else. You smoked while you lived in my house. You think I couldn't smell it on you? Why would you want to smoke now, after everything that you have been through?" She is getting louder and louder. "You are trying to kill yourself, aren't you! YOU are just trying to KILL YOURSELF. If you didn't want me to come to your house, YOU should have just said so. Instead of making excuses about cigarettes."

Didn't I ask her to come by after dinner? Isn't that what I've been trying to do these last five minutes?

There is nothing I can say at this point. She is completely irrational. Out of control. I look over at Jocelyn, who is like a deer caught in the headlights. Though I've told her about Mom's spells, she has never seen my mother like this in person. Let alone in public.

The hospital phone rings, but that doesn't stop my mother's rage, now mixed with sobbing. Jocelyn picks up the phone. I can tell by the bits and pieces that I can hear over my mother's tirade that it is my Dad on the other line.

My Dad is not helpful in these situations involving my Mom. He would rather not deal and wait for things to blow over.

And still my Mom keeps screaming, which makes me want the sweet smoke of a cigarette that much more.

Finally, having screamed herself quiet, she storms out of my room like a tornado of emotion leaving its destruction behind.

Jocelyn stares at me in disbelief. Still shaken and shocked, she finally speaks. "That was ridiculous. She is a complete mess. She needs someone to get her under control."

Sadly, the scene neither shakes me nor surprises me. I have seen my mother like that more times than I care to admit. I don't have time to deal with my Mom's breakdown today. I just want to find Dr. Titleman and go home. Not just for a cigarette but for my sanity.

I get out of bed, and Jocelyn puts her arm around me. "Let me walk, baby," I tell her. "I don't want Dr. Titleman to think I need any assistance."

She lets me go and I confidently walk out the door of Emerson 484. I can see Dr. Titleman standing by the nurses' station, so Jocelyn and I proceed in his direction. His eyes turn to meet mine, and his face shows his disbelief as I march quickly to his side.

"Hi, Dr. Titleman."

"Hello, Matthew. What can I do for you?"

"Can you send me home?"

"Actually, I am writing your prescriptions right now. Go back to your room and gather your belongings. I will be right in to release you and give you your instructions."

"No problem." I give him my biggest smile.

Jocelyn and I walk back to the room and she starts to gather my few belongings. We have two baskets of flowers, a candy basket, and some magazines, but it really isn't too much. I also have the cane that I am debating on whether or not to leave behind.

"Do you think I need the cane?"

"It is up to you," she says, "but I would take it. Just in case."

Dr. Titleman walks in with an orderly, who is pushing a wheelchair.

"Okay, Matthew," he says. "I am going to prescribe you prednisone. Start with 600 milligrams and reduce your consumption by 100 milligrams every three days until you have used all of the pills. Each pill is 100 milligrams, so the first three days take six, the next three days take five and so on. Do you understand?"

"Yes."

"I am also going to prescribe an acid reflux drug to prevent irritation to your stomach lining that you will likely experience on the prednisone. You do not have to change your eating habits for this drug, but I would recommend that you take it daily until you are finished with the prednisone."

"Okay."

"And, finally, I am giving you Roxicet. It's a prescription painkiller for the headaches. Call Dr. Kumar if the headaches do not decrease within the next seven to ten days. If you need any more of the painkillers, call Dr. Kumar, as well."

"Okay."

"The orderly will take you out to your car by wheelchair. Do you have any questions for me?"

"No, Dr. Titleman, but thank you for all of your help over the past couple of days."

"You're welcome, Matthew. Good luck."

He walks out of my room and the orderly assists me into the wheelchair. I take one last, long look around Emerson 484. It is still just a bland white room with a small window. I sigh. I am going home.

Chapter Twenty One - Home at Last

After Jocelyn pulls the car around to the entrance, the orderly loads the three baskets in the back seat and I use my cane to stand up and walk to the passenger door. As I am bending down into the car, I tilt my head as I usually have to do so as not to hit it on the top of the door. I notice how stiff my neck is. Strange. It hasn't been stiff all day. Maybe I've been too consumed with the idea of going home to notice it.

"Jocelyn, I don't feel good. I need to lie down."

She starts the car, the orderly closes the door behind me, and we take off. "You'll be home in one minute, baby," she says. "Don't worry."

"Okay."

I am feeling nauseous. I haven't sat up straight in days. I've been reclining against the raised head of the hospital bed. I realize now that sitting does not feel good at all. I start feeling pressure in my lower back. The nausea increases. And then comes the lightning-strike brain storm.

Jocelyn continues down the road.

"I don't know if I'm going to make it, baby," I groan. "Maybe we should go back."

The headache is blinding me. This is the longest mile of my life.

"We're pulling into the driveway now," she says. The car comes to a stop. "I'm going to go open the door."

"Okay. Hurry!" My head is splitting.

The car door opens. I cannot see through the tears. I bend my neck again to get out of the car, and another huge lightning bolt crashes through my skull. The aftershock reverberates through my entire body.

Jocelyn holds me, and we slowly walk to the door.

The penguin walk is back.

The tears blur everything. I am reaching out with my hands like a blind man with no cane. Jocelyn is saying something. I press onward. We reach the five steps to our house and start to go up. I lean toward the house. Jocelyn gets behind me, puts her hands on my back, and steadies me up the steps.

"We're almost there, baby. You can do it!"

I drop to my knees. I can feel the cold slate of the landing as I crawl through the door Jocelyn has propped open. I inch toward the couch.

My watering eyes are turning to rivers of tears. I can't see the couch, which is directly ahead of me. I bump my head on the glass coffee table and collapse on the floor.

"You okay, baby?"

"No," I gasp.

All she can say is, "Can I do anything for you?"

"I don't know. Just give me a minute on the floor here."

The cold tile feels good against my feverish head. The nausea begins to subside. I look up at the couch and then push myself up on my knees and reach upward. I get a firm grip on the couch on my second try and slowly pull myself up. Once on the couch, I lie on my back and stretch out as far as I can go. I stare straight up toward the ceiling, and then I tilt my head slightly to the left and stare out of the window above the couch. Then, just as suddenly as it came, the storm in my head begins to subside. I lie still, focusing on the pine tree that I can just barely see out the window. Soon the pain is down to bearable. I continue to focus on the outline of my neighbor's pine tree blowing in the wind.

"How are you feeling, baby?" Jocelyn asks.

"I think I'm a little better now. I think I need you to go get those painkillers for me, though."

"Do you need dinner? Something to drink?"

"I can't possibly eat now, but I will take a glass of

water, if you don't mind. Also, could you throw on the TV for me? Put on ESPN."

"Okay, baby. After that, I'm going to run to the drug store to get you your medicine."

She turns on the TV, gets me a glass of water, organizes everything around me, and then leaves. She is gone a few minutes before I realize that this is the perfect opportunity to smoke.

I swing my legs off of the couch and sit up.

No headache.

No stiff neck.

I rise to my feet and grab the cane, which is leaning against the side of the couch. I steady myself on my feet and walk to the door. In a sideways manner, I carefully go down the front steps, facing the house and lowering one foot at a time until I reach the driveway. My pickup truck is only a few feet in front of me. I have no problems reaching the door. But when I open the door and try to climb inside of the truck to sit down, my neck stiffens up again.

Okay, so sitting doesn't work. I'll just stand here and smoke this cigarette like it's a victory cigar.

The stale smoke of the five-day-old cigarette fills my lungs and I cough a little, but I keep smoking. I start to develop that formaldehyde taste in my mouth that I experienced during my spinal tap, but I can't put down the cigarette.

It is absolutely horrible. Why do I miss this feeling?

I flick the cigarette onto the grass and make my way back to the house. The formaldehyde taste begins to grow, and a minute later lightning splits my skull with all the symptoms returning.

I drop to my knees, crawl up the steps, and collapse again onto the cold, hard tile, leaving my feet numbly hanging out the door.

As I lie on the floor, recovering from another violent

headache, I begin to ponder time. From the hospital to my front door is approximately five minutes. From the couch to my truck to smoke is also approximately five minutes. If this trend continues, I have about a five-minute span in which I am able to move around headache free. This already seems inconvenient.

I force my way to the couch and melt down into my comfortable spot with my head and neck propped up on the armrest and my head tilted toward the window. I look out the window at the old pine tree. This is the only position where I don't experience headaches.

I am now a prisoner of the couch.

~~~

Jocelyn walks in. "Matty, you awake?" she whispers.
"Yes, baby."
"I got you all of your stuff."
"Give me a painkiller, please?"
"First, I need you to eat. I got you a small steak and cheese. The medicine has to be taken with food. Can you sit up and eat?"
"I don't know. This is the only position that seems to work. If I move to any other position, I get these crippling headaches."
She looks down sympathetically. "I know but just try"
"Ok."
She goes into the kitchen and puts the sandwich on a plate and cuts it up into bite-sized pieces. Then she comes back and props a pillow behind my back so I can sit up a little. It takes me all of a minute to inhale the sub. I have forgotten how delicious a real sandwich can be.

Jocelyn returns and hands me eight pills. Six are small, the seventh is a large pill that looks like an oversized aspirin, and the eighth is cylindrical. I throw all eight into my mouth at once, drink some water, and swallow hard. Then I slither back down into my comfortable position and gaze up at the old, familiar pine tree. Happily drifting into dreamland.

Chapter Twenty Two - Saturday, May 27

I'm still lying on my couch staring up at the sun. There's no shade on the window. Before my hospital ordeal, Jocelyn ordered some custom shades for this room, but they haven't come in yet. The sun has turned my spot of the living room into a convection oven, and I'm the one cooking in it. Sweating, sticking to the leather of the couch, and too hot to sleep. This is the only spot and position that keeps the spinal headaches at bay, though.

Jocelyn just left to pick up her dad at the airport. With her gone and my current uncomfortable state, there's only one thing to do. Smoke cigarettes.

I'm a little better today. My legs are less stiff, so I have about two more minutes on my feet. This brings me to about seven minutes of freedom before I need to get back to my prison on the couch. My cigarettes are out in my truck. It takes me about three minutes to smoke a cigarette. My flip-flops are at the foot of the couch, and the keys to the truck are in the bowl on the coffee table. I can sneak outside and have two cigarettes without triggering a spinal headache!

As I pull myself up to a sitting position and put on my flip-flops, I notice that sitting is the most uncomfortable position I can be in. Sitting up accelerates the onset of the dreaded symptoms. I grab the keys and force myself up quickly, reaching out for the bookcase to steady myself. Before I know it, I'm at the back door.

Once outside, I take a deep breath of fresh air. I head around the back corner of the house to the driveway where my truck is parked. I reach in, fumble for the glove box, and find the pack of cigarettes. One left. Shit.

I look across the street at the parking lot of the strip mall. I can get a fresh pack at the mini-mart. I think I can walk over there and back again, but that might take about ten minutes. Do I have ten minutes on my feet? I need cigarettes. Is this really even a question?

I flame the last stale smoke and head towards the street. Luckily, out of habit, I grabbed my wallet and keys at the same time, so I don't have to back track to the house and waste precious, headache-free time. More luck. Traffic is light. No problems crossing the street. Despite wearing flip flops, I can navigate down the sidewalk and through the little wooded area to the parking lot and into the store with no problem, either. The store is empty except for the usual elderly clerk. I ask for two packs of smokes and hand over my credit card to pay for them.

I've been gone about five minutes. No headache yet, but my sense of urgency is setting in. I have to get back to the couch soon. The clerk hands me back my card and the two packs of smokes and I quickly exit the store.

I take a moment in front of the store to tear into the new pack and burn a fresh one. It's been like seven or eight minutes now, and I'm not writhing in pain on the ground, but I sure don't want to chance it. Gotta hustle back to the house.

I'm starting to feel dizzy. My seven minutes are long since up. I flick the half-smoked cigarette into the gutter and head inside. I wash my hands at the kitchen sink and then collapse back onto the couch. All told, I've been off the couch for just over ten minutes. Sure, I am dizzy and uncomfortable, but I am not getting another crippling headache. Maybe there is light at the end of the tunnel, after all.

Either way, all this moving around has worn me out. I take a pain pill and assume the position. I may be hot and uncomfortable for now, but the Roxicet will make it all better. I close my eyes and wait for the reinforcements to arrive.

Chapter Twenty Three - Sunday, May 28

I'm standing in front of the mirror for the first time since I left the hospital. I look like a zombie. Still, Jocelyn thinks showering and changing clothes will be good for my well-being. The shower's running and steam is filling the bathroom. Jocelyn helps me undress because I'm not sure I have the stamina. The headaches still have me strung out and weak.

I turn to face the water, but my neck is so incredibly stiff. When I turn, I have to turn my whole body at once. There's also the shame in having another person help me shower, even if that person is my wife. How did I go from so strong, so independent to depending on someone else for even the most rudimentary daily tasks?

Joci's great, though. She has to go back to work today, and now, as soon as she gets home, she's back to caring for me. She helps me into the shower and I lean in under the streaming water. She washes me tenderly with a wash cloth as I close my eyes and let the water permeate my brain.

"Where is your dad?" I ask her.

"He went to Lowe's. He is getting some materials to fix the shed. You've slept so much since he got here yesterday, he figured if you were going to sleep, he might as well do a project."

"A shower is exactly what I needed. Thank you."

"Well, you are definitely getting better. When you first got home, you only had about five minutes on your feet. Now you're up to about ten minutes."

"Yeah, I do feel a bit better."

Just as she says that, however, my body chemistry suddenly changes. The water on my head goes from soothing to painful daggers. I feel my world start to spin and the saliva comes flooding back up in my mouth.

"Jocelyn, I think my ten minutes are up."

"Headache?"

"Yeah. Hurry."

She cuts the water and pulls back the shower curtain. She helps me out of the tub and onto the bathmat. I can no longer stand by myself. I drop to my knees and then lie flat out on the cold bathroom tile floor. She brings out a towel and starts drying me as I lie there, convulsing on the floor.

"Please, baby, make it stop."

Chapter Twenty Four - Friday, June 3

Five days pass. I'm lying on the couch looking at the pine tree above the window. Three pill bottles on the coffee table. A cup of water next to the pills. The light of the TV. A sweat-drenched pillow. Different day. Same day. I feel like Bill Murray in *Groundhog Day*.

The frequency of the headaches has decreased, but my legs are still incredibly weak. I can walk short distances independently, like walking down the hall to the bathroom, but I haven't really tested myself away from the house for any extended length of time. My father-in-law, Jon, has been watching me since Jocelyn returned to work on Monday. For the most part, I've been taking pain pills, sleeping, sneaking cigarettes and going on Dunkin Donut runs. Believe it or not, those runs to Dunkin Donuts are the only times I feel like I can be independent again. I need to branch out and push myself.

Looking up from the couch, I see Jon sitting at the table eating the Dunkin' Donuts breakfast I dragged home earlier this morning in attempt to get my nicotine and coffee fix before everyone woke up. The strain of the mile drive is still too much for my body to take so I collapsed into another Roxi-induced sleep after I arrived home. Jocelyn has already left for work and this is my third day under Jon's care.

"Good morning, Jon."

"Matty, I tell ya," he answers in his usual cheerful tone, "I really appreciate the donuts, but wish you didn't sneak out and drive like that." He gets out of the chair and crosses the room. "I know you want to start doing normal things again, but you still need to rest and recover."

"Yeah. You're right. Sitting in the truck gave me a massive headache. I haven't had one like that in days."

"Well, those are going to take some time to fully go

away but you seem to be getting better each day," Jon adds, focusing on the positive.

"Yeah, Dr. Kumar said it could take awhile."

"Oh, speaking of Dr. Kumar. His office called while you were sleeping. Your test results are going to be in and they want you to come in on Friday the 10th."

Wow. Friday. Seven more days.

In a week, I'll find out what this all means. The physical suffering has been nothing compared to the feeling of not knowing what fate has in store for me. Am I ever going to be the same person again?

~~~

I'm racing down Route 95 toward Providence. Jocelyn has sent Jon and me on an errand to pick up the blinds for the living room windows. The drive is almost an hour away. I have started to wean myself off of the Roxicets, and I'm craving nicotine … A bad combination which is making me feel a bit strung out.

The wind is coming through both windows of the truck. "So," Jon yells above the noise, "are you nervous about seeing the neurologist next Friday?" He sounds like he's giving last-second instructions before a parachute jump.

I'm concentrating on the road. "No. I just want to get it over with." I say matter-of-factly.

He rolls up his window, killing some of the wind noise, but I don't want to engage in conversation. All I want is a cigarette. And to be left alone. I'm sick of talking about my health.

"Hey, would you mind rolling up the window?" he yells.

I grind my teeth as I roll the window up, and then Jon reaches over and turns the radio off. My blood is starting to boil. I want to feel the wind. Listen to music. Be alone. I don't want to revisit the same conversation I've been having over and over and over. But here it is again. All I can do is take a deep breath.

"So," he says, "I've been watching you make great strides during the time I've been here. When I first got here, you were barely mobile. Now you're walking great and not getting the severe headaches." He gives me an optimistic smile. "I think you've made a successful recovery." He pats my shoulder.

I'm not in a good mood, and the nicotine withdrawal makes any physical contact annoying. Even a little pat on the back.

"Does it matter?" My voice is as sour as my mood. "I'm still going to be sick. Twenty eight years old and no future. I mean, what about Jocelyn?"

"What do you mean?"

"I don't want to become a burden on her, man. I promised her that I would provide for her. I promised her that she would be able to stay home and raise our kids. Now I don't feel like I can even promise her a tomorrow."

He looks at me like I'm possessed. "It isn't like you walked out of the house and got hit by a bus," he says, sounding reasonable. "You're going to be fine. Just look at how much progress you've made. I'm real proud of how far you've come just in the short time I've been here. I don't have any question that you'll be back to a hundred percent soon."

Hit by a bus? I can't believe he just pulled that old cliché out on me. I've spent the better half of the last month crippled from the waist down and may or may not have a chronic illness. Being hit by a bus would be an upgrade at this point.

"No, Jon. It is like I got hit by a bus, but it didn't kill me. It just crippled me for a while. Now I have to wait and see if it will cripple me for life."

He crosses his arms, looking away from me and at the scenery out the window. "Now that's just crazy talk. You need to think about all the good things in your life. Be positive."

"Excuse my French, but I'm sick of being Mr. Fucking Positive! I may have some disease that there is no cure for! I may not be able to have kids, and if I have kids I may not be able to fucking play with them! Jocelyn may have to work for the rest of her fucking life while I fucking putt around in some fucking wheelchair! Who knows if I'll even be fucking coherent or not! You get me now?! I got fucking hit by the fucking bus!"

An awkward silence fills the truck.

Finally he says, "You're swerving a bit here. Just calm down and concentrate on the road, okay?"

"What are you scared of?" I mutter. "Crashing into a bus?"

"Listen. I wish I never said anything about the damn bus, okay? Get over it!"

Now he's becoming huffy. I'm just so strung out. I don't mean to take it out on him. He's been such a great help in my recovery. I change my tack.

"Jon, listen, I don't mean to take this out on you. I'm just scared. I needed to vent."

"I know you do, guy." He taps my shoulder again. "I'm not taking this personally. I know you're scared. Hell, anyone in your position would be scared. Even me. Life as you know it is probably about to change."

Well, that's an understatement, I think. "I know, I know." I look away from the road for a second. "I've come far in a week. I guess I just never thought I would be in this kind of position. Not at this age. I feel like there's so much left for me to do."

"I wouldn't think that you'd be the type of person to pack it in and give up on the world," he says. "You like to prove people wrong. So prove people wrong about this. You just need to focus and overcome this. Like you have everything else in your life."

We have somehow arrived at the store. I pull into a parking space and reflect on the ride for a moment. "Yeah. Hey, sorry about blowing up on you back there. I feel like a jerk."

"That's my job." He smiles at me again. "You aren't a jerk. You're just scared. That's completely normal."

Nothing feels normal at anymore.

Chapter Twenty Five - The Diagnosis

I am in the waiting room of Dr. Kumar's office, sitting in the same chair and flipping through the same outdated *Sports Illustrated* as nearly a month ago. The waiting room is still crowded and the doctor is still running late. It is déjà vu all over again. The difference with this and my initial visit is that a crowd is now joining me and Jocelyn. My Dad, Mom and father-in-law are all here to find out my diagnosis. Oh, and I am walking more normally this time.

Jon and my Dad are talking, Jocelyn is flipping through an outdated gossip magazine, and Mom is trying to get me to make eye contact with her. I don't want to. She looks like she hasn't slept and has been crying. She has no doubt been burdening herself with all the possible "what if" scenarios for this appointment. Seeing her act so nervous makes me nervous. I am trying to focus on the magazine, but negative thoughts are creeping into my mind.

The door opens and Dr. Kumar motions to us. We all stand up together. As I walk over to Dr. Kumar, he examines my every step.

"Hello, Matthew"

We shake hands.

"Hi, Dr. Kumar. Long time, no see."

"Riiiiight. Well, it is good to see that you are walking better."

"Still not quite a hundred percent, but I'm sure getting there." I pause and gesture at the mob standing behind me. "Do you mind if my family comes in with me?"

"No problem at all." Dr. Kumar smiles and ushers them through the door. "Good to see you all."

After making introductions, I follow Dr. Kumar down the hall, and everyone follows me in a line. The hall is quiet and dimly lit. I feel Dr. Kumar still scrutinizing my every step as we enter his office. I take the same seat in front of Dr. Kumar's desk that I'd taken a month earlier. Jocelyn sits in the chair next to me and my Mom, Dad, and Jon stand behind us.

Dr. Kumar takes his seat at his desk, opens my file, taking a deep breath.

The blinds are pulled so that Dr. Kumar is sitting in shadows behind his desk. He leans back in his oversized office chair and waits for us to settle in. But I have waited long enough.

Making eye contact with me, Dr. Kumar leans forward in his chair. "I'm sorry it took so long to get the data back," he says. "We send the blood work and spinal fluid to an outside lab for analysis, and it generally takes a couple of weeks before the results are available. I know you have all been waiting patiently for the results, and I thank you for that."

He stands up and puts my MRI films on a whiteboard, then turns on a fluorescent light to illuminate the pictures. This is the first time that I am seeing my brain and while I might normally be fascinated by the pictures, I just want to hear what they found. "Well, Matthew, the MRI's revealed multiple lesions on your brain and spine. The active lesion is on the spine right here," he picks up a laser pointer and circles a white splotch on one of the photographs, "is the most likely the cause of the Transverse Myelitis."

I'm not sure what exactly he is pointing at but as he talks, he also points to several different areas in some of my brain pictures with similar splotches.

"I then needed to do the additional testing of the blood and spinal fluids before I could make an accurate diagnosis," he continues.

He flicks off the light behind the MRI photos and returns to his seat. He leans forward and looks me square in the eyes, "Matthew, there is no easy way to say this." He pauses, "You have Multiple Sclerosis."

The room is quiet. Jocelyn reaches across her chair, grabs my hand and squeezes it tight, but I am numb. I stare forward not wanting to see the expressions on the others' faces.

"To expand further," the doctor adds, "given the location of your lesions on both your brain and your spine, you exhibit the profile of relapsing remitting MS, or RRMS."

Jocelyn squeezes my hand tighter. I finally look to her and she mouths, "It's okay" but I see the fear in her eyes. I try to gain control of my senses, but my vision seems blurry and my hearing impaired.

Dr. Kumar clears his throat. "Here is the good news, Matthew. There are several treatment options available today that help slow the progression of the disease."

Good news? How is anything he is telling me right now good news? I am going from confused to mad. I feel rage in the pit of my stomach. I want to stand up and smash something. How can I possibly have MS? The only thing I know about MS is that it doesn't end well. Not well at all.

"So how long do I have before I am going to be in a wheelchair?" I say under my breath.

Jocelyn squeezes my hand again.

Dr. Kumar assures the room, "Multiple Sclerosis research and treatment has come a long way in the past ten years. There are a lot of resources that you have as an MS patient today that can help you lead a normal life. The National MS Society, for example."

This still isn't sinking in. This can't be happening. I don't want to believe this is really happening. I feel like I am watching a scene from a movie. And I am the tragic main character.

"Dr. Kumar," I finally say, "this doesn't make any sense to me. I mean, before this happened with my legs, I never experienced any symptoms before. No numbness, no tingling, no nothing."

There is a collective head nod and grumble behind me. Maybe this is all a big mistake.

Dr. Kumar settles us back down. "Matthew, you have probably experienced minor symptoms over the years and passed them off as something else. Fatigue, for instance."

Now a collective groan and rumblings of how much I've enjoyed sleep throughout my life.

Dr. Kumar tries to quiet the chatter and takes the floor again. "MS symptoms can manifest in a variety of ways which differ from individual and range in severity."

Enough with the MS101 already. I need to get out of here. And fast.

Sensing my growing anxiety with the situation, Jocelyn asks, "So, what is the treatment option that you recommend for Matt?"

Dr. Kumar nods at Jocelyn. "Currently, there are four injectable treatments available. We call the treatments the ABC's and R: Avonex, Betaseron, Copaxone, and Rebif. I have patients doing well on each of these treatments, and I would be comfortable prescribing any one of these to you. I want to give you information packets on all four treatments so that you can make an informed decision on your own. The biggest difference between these treatments is the frequency of dosage. For instance, the Copaxone is once a day, whereas the Avonex is once a week. Betaseron and Rebif are administered roughly every other day. Take this information home and make an informed decision as to the treatment path you would like to take."

Shots? This is getting out of hand. I don't want to get poked every day for the rest of my life.

"What about children?" Jocelyn softly asks.

"This shouldn't affect his ability to have children at all." Dr. Kumar assures her.

I feel like the walls are closing in. I need to get out of

here before I have a meltdown.

"Is that it, Dr. Kumar? I want to get going."

I can feel my Dad's glare of disapproval on my back.

"So who would give Matt these shots?" Jocelyn asks

No one is listening to me. I am done. I want to go. There is nothing that this doctor is going to tell me to make it all right. But the MS101 lecture continues.

Dr. Kumar continues, "Typically the patient administers the shots themselves to their upper thigh or arm. With all the treatments, a nurse will come to your home and teach you how to properly administer the medication."

I shake my head. "No. There's no way I'm touching a needle. I can't do it. I won't."

"If you are not comfortable," the doctor replies, "perhaps your wife can do it for you. But I would recommend you start treatment immediately."

Jocelyn sits up straight and nods her head to Dr. Kumar ready to do whatever it takes.

As Dr. Kumar continues explaining the drug options, my family, behind me, starts buzzing about the treatment options. I am surrounded. I don't want to hear any of it. Every word feels like an assault. I am ready to just stand up and walk out of here.

Then I look over at Jocelyn again. She gives me a brave, reassuring smile. But I know that her heart is broken into a million different pieces. She gently motions me to listen to the doctor. Despite all my reservations, I know I am going to have to start a treatment regimen. And she is going to have to help me do it.

She addresses Dr. Kumar. "Did I hear you say that there was a once-a-week treatment?"

"Yes. Avonex is administered once a week."

"Is Avonex something that would work well for Matt? Once a week seems a lot better than every day."

"Like I said, I would feel comfortable prescribing any

of the ABCR's to Matthew. Please take the information and read it over. For instance, Copaxone is every day, but it is a smaller subcutaneous needle. Patients typically report little to no side effects, whereas Avonex is a longer intramuscular needle and the concentrated, once a week, dose can lead to flu-like symptoms. It is important to weigh all of your options."

Without thinking, I blurt out, "Dr. Kumar, for me, I don't want to do shots. If I have to do shots, I want to do the least amount possible. I think I'll try the Avonex."

Dr. Kumar pauses and looks me in the eye. "I know that I have given you a lot of information here today. I want you to take home all of the pamphlets and look them over. Each has different pros and cons. I really want you to make an informed decision."

"Okay, I get it. I'll go home and think it over. Dr. Kumar, thank you for everything." I stand up and shake his hand.

"Sorry I had to deliver the news, Matt. I know this has been a difficult process. Just remember that there are tremendous strides being made with MS."

I nod, thank him again, then turn and head toward the door. Jocelyn gathers up all the drug information and puts it in her purse. The parents stay behind, asking Dr. Kumar questions. Everyone seems to be in a positive place, believing, like Dr. Kumar, that MS is manageable and I can still have a normal life. Everyone but me.

~~~

After some awkward silence leaving Dr. Kumar's office, we all congregate in front of my Dad's car in the parking lot. I hate the looks of pity and sadness masked by fake smiles. I really need a change of scenery.

I finally say, "Hey, thanks for coming with me but I

need to go now." And start walking towards my car not wanting to be held up any longer by anything or anyone.

My Dad calls out, "Matt, I have to take your Mom to work now but you want to meet at Denly's for some dinner?"

This is by far the best thing anyone has said to me all day. Denly's is a hole in the wall pizza shop down the street from my Grandmother's house that my family has gone to every week since I can remember. If anything is going to help me deal right now, it is good pizza and cold beer. "Yeah," I say, "we'll meet you over there."

During the drive, Jon and Jocelyn keep up the positive talk. I stay quiet.

As we make our way to Denly's, we drive past my Aunt and Grandmother's house. I wonder if my Dad told my Aunt yet. That first night in the emergency room, before the doctors even ran a test, she told Jocelyn that she thought it was MS. She had been through it before with her sister, Loretta, and knew the symptoms of the disease all too well, I guess.

When we arrive, we get a booth near the bar. I squeeze in and take a seat near the window, so I can watch traffic and avoid talking about my condition. Jocelyn squeezes in next to me, and Jon sits on the other side. I am too big for the booth. My knees hit the table, which is tight up against me.

"Peter!" voices from the bar call as my Dad walks in like Norm from *Cheers*. My Dad stops at the bar and socializes with a couple of guys before making his way over to the table.

Once he sits down next to Jon, a waitress comes over.

"What can I get you, Pete?"

"I'll have a Miller Lite."

"Okay. Everyone else?"

"I'll have a Stella and a frost mug," I say.

"I'll just have a draft," Jon says.

"And I'll have a glass of Chardonnay," Jocelyn adds.

We order for a couple of pizzas, as well. I keep looking

out the window and zone out into a distant place. Moments later, the beers arrive and I snap back to reality. I pour my Stella into the frosted mug in front of me and take a long drink.

The table is making small talk but it all sounds like white noise to me.

I take another series of gulps, finishing the first beer. I motion to the waitress with the empty glass. She gives me the nod.

I stare out the window.

My second beer arrives. I am already feeling a little loose from the first one. I take another big gulp and listen to my Dad talk about the benefits of vitamins. Then the talk finally finds its way back over to me.

"So," Dad says, "how are you doing with all this, Matt? I know they say that there's no proof that it's genetic, but it's always something I feared when I looked at my sister. You were just a little boy when she died. As I watched her dying, I just didn't want you to end up like that. I didn't want any of my kids to go through what she went through. Your mother and I kind of feel responsible for this."

"It's not your fault, Dad."

"Yeah, Peter," says Jocelyn. "It could have happened to any one of your kids."

Dad turns and looks at me, all serious, "Well, if any one of my kids was gonna get sick, I'm glad it is you."

What the hell? What does he even mean by that?

"I guess I'm glad it could be me, too, Dad." I say sarcastically. I take another series of gulps. He misses my sarcasm, of course, and my mind is still racing to process what he means. I chug the rest of my second beer and slam the empty mug down. I wave for a third one.

Dad finally figures out that I am not taking his comment well. "Slow down, will ya?" He takes a drink of his beer. "I didn't mean it like that." He is back-pedaling now.

"Don't be so sensitive. I meant that of all my kids, you're the one who can handle it."

My third beer arrives. I drink it. Somehow, Dad's explanation, which makes more sense to me, still hurts. The pizzas arrive, along with my fourth beer. Having had three in under twenty minutes, I am pretty buzzed.

"You know what, Dad? Maybe I can't handle this one."

Chapter Twenty Six - Saturday, June 11

I hear the back door open and shut. My eyes open to catch a new day's light spilling in from space between the drawn shade and windowsill. I have a mild headache from last night's alcohol, but other than that, I feel fine. After Denly's, we came home and I went right to bed. Now I can hear the new doors to our remodeled shed in the back yard open and some banging like someone is moving something. Jon must be heading out for his morning bike ride.

I'm wide awake, lying on my side under the covers. I've got a pillow wedged in between my knees to keep the bones from mashing together. I haven't been this comfortable since before I lost feeling in my legs. Maybe it was the booze, but for the first time in a long time, I slept peacefully last night.

But now my mind starts working again. The tranquility of night surrenders to the reality of the day. And my reality has changed dramatically.

Hi, my name is Matt and I have Multiple Sclerosis. It still hasn't fully sunk in yet. With the numbness gone from my lower half, I can feel warmth through my whole body, like my nerves are reconnecting. I'm starting to feel like … like I'm not really … not really damaged.

I'm not even fighting the urge for my morning smoke. And the coffee can wait, too. The urge to sneak out and hide my bad habit is gone, if only for this moment. The window is open a crack, and a breeze drifts into the room.

I take a deep breath and hold it. Jocelyn is facing me, smiling in her sleep. I brush her blonde hair away from her eyes. I'm gazing at her sleeping peacefully by my side, as if last night was just any other night. She's still the same girl I met all those years ago in Arizona. The knockout blonde who climbed a fence to make out with me in the pool under the bright Tempe moon. That same girl whose love has never wavered for one second, in my darkest hour, even when everyone else around her was losing it. I think that kind of silent strength can be taken for granted.

But I'm not the same boy I was two months ago. Probably never will be the same again. I can't take things for granted anymore.

I just want to be lying with her at this moment. Enjoying:

The breeze.

The toasty sunlight.

My erect penis?

Oh, my God.

MY ERECT PENIS!

I can't even remember the last time I had an erection. It had to be well over a month ago. The last remaining MS hostage has been released. Jocelyn needs to see this. I shake her shoulder.

"Jocelyn"

"Mmmmmmff?"

I kiss her forehead. She opens her eyes and looks at me. I don't hesitate. I bring my lips to hers and close my eyes. Our lips tingle as they touch.

Her eyes pop open.

"You know how I was having a problem down there?" I whisper and point towards my groin.

"Uh huh." She's becoming more awake.

"Well ... it's working again!" I say with excitement.

With that, she reaches into my boxers, "It is working! Too bad my dad's next door," she whispers.

I can't help but grin. "I actually just heard him take off on his bike ride. He's usually gone an hour or so. We have plenty of time."

We start kissing again. Her mouth becomes wetter, she opens it and begins moving her tongue over mine. I reach under her loose cotton T-shirt and tickle the soft skin of her belly with the tips of my fingers, and warm goose bumps dance across her skin. I begin kissing her neck. I love the taste of her skin in the morning.

She runs her hand down my bare chest and over my boxer shorts. She's really awake now. I can tell she's ready.

My right hand slowly traces the curves of her body as we look deep into each others' eyes, as if we never thought this moment would happen again. Not a word is said, but we both understand. With all we've been through and all the challenges that still remain, here we are. Still together. Still madly in love. This is our moment.

She pulls away from me and sits up. My eyes follow her. Then she looks back at me, smiles, and lifts her T-shirt over her head, exposing her perfect breasts. She tosses her shirt over the side of the bed and lunges at me. I pull her back down to me and start kissing and licking her breasts. My hand creeps toward her panty line.

My index finger is massaging her in a slow circular motion. She begins to squirm as her juices start flowing, and she bites down hard on her lip as she moans. I suck on her breast while my fingers are working deeper into her pleasure center.

"I missed you," she murmurs. She pulls my hands away. "I want you inside me."

She is lying on her back. I move on top of her. She helps guide me between her legs. I feel her warmth against me and my every nerve tingle as she lets me in.

Oh, God! For a whole month, I thought I would never feel these sensations again.

I push forward and back, feeling her warm lubrication flowing up and down on me. We begin to rock back and forth, our bodies in tune to our primal desires. The pace quickens. The bed squeaks louder. She slams her eyes shut and drags her nails against my back. She bites my ear. We rock back and forth, harder and harder.

Quicker and quicker. Faster and harder. Until—sweet release.

We collapse into each other, the beads of sweat on her neck glistening in the new day's light. She lets out a satisfied sigh, and I bring my lips to her neck again and kiss her gently.

She doesn't say anything, but just pulls my head against her bare chest. I feel her heartbeat as she holds me tight. We lie together in silence, enjoying the warmth of each other and the new day's sun.

Chapter Twenty Seven - Being Followed by a Moon Shadow

It is a beautiful early summer New England day, the kind of day that makes you forget the long, hard winter you've just lived through. The temperature is in the mid-seventies, the sun is warm on my face, the colors of spring are in bloom, and I have just made love to my wife. So why am I feeling … restless? Maybe it is because I am still trying to digest what I learned yesterday at Dr. Kumar's office.

I don't even want to think about it. I just want to drive.

I cruise the windy back roads of our town, slowing down a bit as I pass the pond where my Grandfather took me fishing when I was a boy. That was the only time I have ever gone fishing. I caught one that day. A small, ugly catfish, but to hear my Grandpa tell it, it was Moby Dick.

My truck climbs a hill, on top of which sits my Grandmother's little white house with green shutters. I pull up along the sidewalk. No one is home. I get out and stand on the sidewalk, sparking a smoke, then leaning up against my truck and gazing at the house.

My family has called this house home ever since they got off the boat from Italy in the early nineteen hundreds. At one time, there was a magnificent garden in back. My Grandfather used to let me help tend to the garden when I was a boy. When he got tired of me and my little plastic rake, he would put me on the sidewalk with a box of tomatoes to sell. I don't recall ever selling a tomato to anyone, but he convinced me that was the best way to help, so I always sat there for hours with my box of tomatoes. My Aunt would always give me a Buster Bar from Dairy Queen as a reward. That's how I knew I was helping.

Tossing the cigarette butt into the street, I get back into the truck and kick it into first gear, continuing on down the street, making a right and then a quick left.

Ah, there it is. The small ranch house where I was born. It looks tiny, even in comparison to the small ranch house I have now. My memories of this house are still foggy. Cracked sidewalk in front. Small green lawn. I remember a big sandbox out back where I played. There is now a fence surrounding the yard.

This was my home until I was five years old. Now someone else lives here. Ironically, someone has installed a handicap ramp leading to the front door. The sight of the ramp sends unsettling chills up my spine. I jam the truck back into first and squeal out of there.

Now my head-clearing drive is starting to bother me. These places of my youth that are supposed to comfort me are contributing to my anxiety. I am rattled, but determined to find some comfort on this drive.

Where am I going, anyway? Now I cross over to the bordering town where I lived most of my childhood. Soon I pull out onto Main Street and pass the elementary school. Since my days there, they've added on to that old, red-brick school.

I turn the radio off. The only thing I want to hear is the wind. I continue on, recalling various details of my youth. I am driving almost unconsciously but suddenly the forest ends and I see the ocean.

A cement beach wall protects the sand below and old, weather-worn stairs lead down to this jewel of a beach. I pull into the lot above the wall and park my truck up against it, facing the ocean. Then I turn the engine off and look out at the water. I can hear the waves crashing and the wind singing through my open windows. I look over toward the rocks and see the little cove where I used to escape to when I was a kid. It is this little inlet in between boulders that always has a pool of warm water cupped inside it.

The wind sings and the waves crash.

Singing and crashing.

Over and over.

I am mesmerized

And then …

Something way deep inside my head starts up. A little melody. Then it turns into a song bouncing around the inside of my head. It is a familiar song, but I can't quite remember what it is. I can't catch the whole tune.

Bit by bit, it comes to me, and soon I am sitting there, looking out at the water and humming the tune. I am remembering now. It is a song from my childhood. It is familiar, but still distant. I can almost hear the acoustic guitar riffs. They get clearer. Then almost subconsciously I start to sing the refrain.

"I'm being followed by a Moonshadow. Moonshadow. Moonshadow."

Cat Stevens' "Moonshadow"? Now I know I am crazy. Of all the songs in the world, of all the thoughts I could be thinking, why am I hearing "Moonshadow" in my head?

I try to remember more of the lyrics. There has to be a reason I am singing this song. It isn't like I am a particularly big Cat Stevens fan. This is a song from my Dad's generation. Why can't I stop hearing this song in my head?

I fire up the engine to my truck and throw it in reverse. BEEP!

"Sorry!" I yell.

I look back to see that I almost jackknifed the side of an oncoming car. The driver flicks me off, but I don't care. My Dad has some of Cat's CDs. I have to get to my parents house and find this song. I need to hear all the lyrics right now.

I pull into my parents' driveway, open the driver's side door and leave the truck running as I race through the front door. My parents are both sitting at the kitchen table as I rush past them.

"Hey Dad, are your CDs still downstairs?" I yell as I run to the basement.

"Yeah, what do you need?" he answers from the top of the stairs.

"I need your Cat Steven's CD!" I yell back.

I walk around the corner and open the walk-in closet that stores the surround-sound to the TV.

Aha.

The crate of CDs is on the bottom shelf. I pull them out, sneezing from the dust. There must be two hundred CDs in the box. I drop down on the floor and start pouring through them. It's a 1970's flashback. The Eagles. James Taylor. Boston. Led Zeppelin.

Finally. I come to the CD I am looking for. I pick it up and stare at the cover. Cat Stevens' *Greatest Hits*.

I flip it over and scan the list of songs. There it is, song number five.

"Moonshadow."

I fly back up the stairs clutching the CD in my hand. My parents are back at the kitchen table, staring at me with a dumbfounded look.

"What do you want a Cat Stevens' CD for?" Dad asks, furrowing his brow.

"I have no idea. Thanks for the CD. I'll talk to you guys later." I respond as I rush back out the door and into my running truck.

I hop into the truck and burn rubber as I back up out of the driveway. I pull into the street and fumble with the CD case. I get the disc into the CD player as quickly as I can and forward to song five.

"Moonshadow."

The acoustic guitars at the beginning of the song resonate through cabin of my truck. Then Cat's voice booms through the speakers. As I head home, I concentrate on the lyrics.

Oh, if I ever lose my legs... Hey, that just happened to me! I try to focus on the song.

If I ever lose my eyes...If I ever lose my mouth.... If I ever lose my hands...

An eerie chill runs through my entire body. This song is talking about all of the things MS can do. Losing my vision, speech, hands, and legs. This song is a glimpse into my future of what horrible fate has in store for me! I start to panic. Maybe if I listen to the song again it won't be so bad.

I stop and replay the track.

I'm being followed by a Moonshadow. Moonshadow. Moonshadow.

Then it hits me like a ton of bricks. There is no mistaking this coincidence. Moonshadow. Moon. Shadow. M. S. My heart sinks.

I am being followed by a Moon Shadow named Multiple Sclerosis. My Moon Shadow is going ravage my body leaving me a crippled version of myself!

As I pull into the driveway, I see Jocelyn and Jon's silhouettes in the window. I pop the CD out of the player and shove it under my seat. I feel defeated and weak. All I want to do is lie down and hid from the world. Hide from the moonshadow that is following me.

Chapter Twenty Eight - Thursday, July 14th 2005

I haven't really left the house since my drive down memory lane. Jon left a couple days ago to go home. Jocelyn is finishing up the school year. I lie on the couch wallowing in self-pity and watching *Sports Center* loops. Life feels far from normal.

A visiting nurse came to the house yesterday to teach me how to inject myself with my new weekly treatment. She had me practice on oranges. I couldn't even do that. My hands were shaky and I grew sick to my stomach at the thought of stabbing myself every week in my thighs or arms. Sensing that I was completely incompetent of injecting myself, she switched gears and focused on teaching Jocelyn how to administer the medication. I could tell that Jocelyn was equally as horrified at the thought of stabbing a needle in me but she didn't protest and took her new role as nursemaid seriously, focusing on every detail of the instructions that the nurse gave her.

Today is going to be the true test- my first injection. No doctors, no nurse. Just me, Jocelyn and an imposing inch and a quarter needle.

The medicine has been sitting on the kitchen counter for an hour or so. Each time I enter and exit the kitchen my eyes are drawn to this humongous needle. I feel like a complete burden to Jocelyn having her administer this shot. If it were up to me, I would not go on any medication at all but I know that would upset Jocelyn even more.

It is dinner time but I'm not hungry. I want to take my shot and go to bed. The anxiety of this moment is eating at me.

"Let's get it over with." I say out of the blue. I go into

the kitchen and pull out the kitchen chair closest to the window and kitchen counter so that Jocelyn can have easy access.

"Ok," Jocelyn says as she walks over to the kitchen sink and starts meticulously washing her hands.

As she approaches me, she takes a deep breath. She pushes the leg of my running shorts up slightly to better access my thigh muscle. She then takes an alcohol wipe and rubs it in a circular motion over my thigh. Using the wipe as a fan, she gently blows on my thigh to dry the alcohol. Then she opens the needle package and attaches the needle to the medicine vial. After a brief struggle she takes off the cap.

"The nurse said that we need to get the bubble out," she says coaching herself as she flicks the vial and depresses the plunger shooting medicine in the air.

"Check you out, Nurse Joci" I say in my best positive voice.

"Are you ready?" she asks.

Our eyes lock. The unspoken truth is that neither of us is ready. This is a part of the journey that neither one of us could have predicted. It is tearing me apart that my wife has to become my nurse this young in life.

"Let's do it." I say.

"I'm just going to plunge it straight down like the nurse said. It's going to be quick." She says, reassuring me and herself at the same time.

I gaze out into the back yard and over the fence. The summer sun is glaring off the neighbor's trampoline where their kids are bouncing, laughing and having fun.

"Ok, I'm going to do it." Jocelyn says after a deep breath.

"It's fine Joci, go ahead."

The next thing I feel is the plunge of a needle deep into the meat of my thigh. A sting overcomes my body as cold medicine enters my muscle.

She exhales deeply, "Are you alright?"

"You did good baby."

"I'm going to take it out." She says seeming relieved it's almost over.

I turn from looking out the window and examine the needle in my leg. She is holding it with a strong, steady hand. It twangs and I flinch as she starts to pull it out.

The needle exits my leg and with it a geyser of blood shoots into the air spewing over six inches above my leg. Jocelyn freezes at the sight.

"Don't just stand there!!! DO SOMETHING!!!" I exclaim.

Jocelyn snaps out of it and grabs some gauze. She applies gauze to the geyser suppressing the mighty stream.

We look at each other in disbelief.

"Let me get a band-aid, hold this." Jocelyn puts my hand on the gauze and grabs the band-aid off of the counter.

"That was crazy." She says shaking her head, still in shock.

It seems that the more days that have passed since my diagnosis, the worse things have gotten. I hardly recognize myself any more, let alone my life. I can't imagine getting this shot every week for the rest of my life. Is that really living? It sure as hell doesn't feel like it tonight.

~~~

We are sitting on the couch watching the TV. That's when the chills set in. All of a sudden a strong fever overcomes me. My skin is on fire. My body starts to shake from extreme chills.

"Jocelyn help!" I cry out. "I feel sick."

"Here drink some water." She grabs a glass of water and brings it to my lips. "This will help."

I try to force it down, but can't.

"I need to get to bed."

Jocelyn helps me up. I am blinded by the flu symptoms and feel incredibly weak. The last time my walking was this bad was when I was recovering.

I climb into bed and throw every blanket over my body.

"I'm freezing." I say, shaking inaudibly.

Jocelyn rushes to get another blanket. The fever is aching every inch of my body and at the injection site is a deep, stabbing pain. I feel tears rolling down my scalding face, turning to steam as they fall.

Jocelyn returns with a blanket. She kisses my forehead.

"You're on fire." She says. "You're all sweaty, too. Do you think it's the medicine?"

I can't talk, I am shaking too hard focusing on the fever.

"I'll let you rest up and get some sleep. It's your birthday tomorrow. We're going to try to go up your parents' and have a party, ok?"

I still can't talk. I don't want a stupid birthday party. What am I celebrating exactly?

"Ok, Matty? You gonna make it?"

"Love you" I manage through chattering teeth.

"Love you, too." She says and leaves the room as I drift into sleep to wrestle my fever.

Chapter Twenty Nine - Friday, July 15 - Happy Birthday!!!

Today I turn 29. I am lying in the cool dewy grass behind my house, sneaking a cigarette and feeling the sun rise. I barely slept last night because of the fever and the body aches that hurt down to my bones. I am exhausted and nauseous and could care less about any kind of celebration. I haven't seen or spoken to most of these people who are going to be at the party since my diagnosis. The only thing that could be worse today than this birthday party is a potential pity party in my honor. I am better off staying at home today so I don't have to talk about how I feel or listen to unsolicited advice about MS "cures" from well-intentioned people without medical degrees. And I definitely don't want to see the looks of concern in peoples' eyes when they come up to me and say in their Polly positive voices, 'Hey, you are going to be just fine.' Truth is no one knows if I will be fine and I certainly don't feel fine.

Then I think about Jocelyn. Not only has all of this been hard on me, but probably equally as hard on her. Only four years ago were we married and now we are already testing the in sickness and in health vow. Now, she is going to be expected to stick a needle in my leg every week of her life for the foreseeable future. She has remained the rock during all of this when everyone around me has fallen apart. Maybe I should attend my party today, just to get Jocelyn out of the house and enjoy a break from babysitting me.

I finally muster up the energy to shower- something I haven't done in more than a couple days now. My skin is broken out and pale and my hair is matted to my head. If I don't want people talking about me being sick, I better try to look a little better. Showering depletes me of any energy I have but at least I look presentable now. I throw on my favorite polo shirt and khaki shorts and meet Jocelyn in the family room.

"You look cute," Jocelyn says with a smile.

"Thanks. Ready to get this over with?" I ask.

"I'm ready if you are"

The four mile ride to my parents' house is silent. I look out the window into the old neighborhoods of my youth feeling more distant from those days than ever before. As we pull into the driveway, I scan the parked cars to identify all the guests in attendance. My cousin, Petey, and his family are here. My Aunt is here, too. So far, only immediate family. This does little to ease my anxiety, though.

"We're not going to stay long, Jocelyn," I say with the car idling in the driveway.

"We'll just do what you think you can handle," she responds.

"I didn't sleep well last night, I'm still feeling sick from the medicine and my legs are weak," I start to explain.

"Everyone at the party knows you're sick, Matt. Why are you worried?"

"I really don't want to have the same conversation over and over. I can't even wrap my head around all of this yet, let alone answer a million questions. I just don't..."

Jocelyn cuts me off, "Matt, it's your birthday. There will be cake and presents. You don't have to talk about anything that you don't want to. The minute it becomes too much, we will just leave. Ok?"

Before I can answer, she is already out of the car. She must really need to get out the house because I have never seen her more determined to go to a party. Jocelyn opens the passenger side of the car and helps me up. My walking is still not back to hundred percent and I am certainly having problems getting in and out of vehicles. As I limp towards the house, I notice people staring out the window, waiting for me. I pull open the front door.

"HAPPY BIRTHDAY!!!" they all exclaim and break into the song.

As they sing, I make my way to the kitchen table where a pineapple upside down cake displays the number twenty nine in burning candles. The song ends and I blow out the candles. Everyone cheers.

"Wow! Right to cake, huh?" I ask.

"We didn't know how you were feeling," my Mom says.

After I make my quick rounds of saying "hello" and "thanks for coming," I plop myself down in a chair waiting for my slice of cake to be served.

Instead of cake, though, Jocelyn brings me a present. She is grinning from ear to ear.

"Here, we want you to open this before you eat the cake," she says as she hands me the gift.

Without unwrapping it, I know it is a book. The size, shape and weight all make it obvious. It is probably some self-help book for people with MS or a holistic, "eat these leaves and you'll be cured" type of book. Either way, I am not much in the mood for reading. However from the anticipating eyes glaring at me at the table, I can tell that they really want me to open this book.

I tear it open and to my disbelief, it is a book about Soft-Coated Wheaten Terriers. It takes a second to compute in my brain.

"Does this mean what I think it does?" I ask.

"Why don't you open the next present?" Jocelyn says beaming as she hands me a smaller package.

I don't waste any time tearing into the second present. Inside is a small orange dog collar. I am in shock and overwhelmed. I look up to Jocelyn to give me an answer.

Jocelyn puts her hand on my knee and looks me in the

eye, "Yes Matt, we're finally getting your puppy."

I am still speechless but the room bursts into commotion. Everyone is talking excitedly among themselves. Camera flashes are blinding me and people are calling out for me to smile and hold up the book. I want to be elated and jump up and down but my heart sinks instead. I just started to regain functionality of my legs and I am not too stable on my feet. Plus, I have been diagnosed with a chronic illness that they don't have a cure for. How am I supposed to take care of and walk a dog? As everyone around me is celebrating, I prepare myself to tell Jocelyn that I am so thankful for this gift but the timing isn't right for me to accept it.

Then, my eyes land on Jocelyn. She is so excited about the puppy and telling my family members all of the details of her covert operation to surprise me with the perfect puppy. Her eyes tell the entire story. I can see at this moment that she needs me to have the puppy more than I ever wanted to get a puppy before in my life.

I grab her with a tear welling up in my eyes and I whisper, "Thank you. I love you."

"I love you, too," she says still beaming with joy over the surprise.

"So, when do we get this puppy?" I ask, still nervous about the prospect.

"He was born on Memorial Day," she says, "so the breeder said we can pick him up on July 30th. We're lucky. The mom had six puppies and five of them are girls. We prepaid, so we have the pick of the litter and will get the only male."

As she talks about the breeder and everything, I am fixated on the birthday.

"Did you say the puppies were born on Memorial Day?"

"Yeah," she says as she continues her story.

Memorial Day. Zack.

"Zack died Memorial Day four years ago. I was always upset that you never got to meet him and that I never got a chance to say goodbye," I say interrupting the conversation again.

"Maybe this puppy is a gift from Zack, too," Jocelyn adds with a smile.

"Yeah, maybe it is." I start to think back on how Zack would get away and I would have to chase him down the street. "It would be just like him to make me get up and walk when I don't want too."

Thanks Zack. Maybe there is reason to celebrate this birthday after all.

Chapter Thirty - Saturday, July 30

It is a gorgeous Massachusetts summer day. The sun is shining bright and the temperature is in the mid-80's with a low breeze and low humidity. The weather is perfect but I am all nerves about picking up our new puppy. I still have doubts about my ability to own a dog right now.

"I'm so excited! I can't wait to meet him," Jocelyn says enthusiastically.

It is funny to me because up until this point, Jocelyn has thought the timing was wrong for us to get a dog. Every time I wanted to get a dog, Jocelyn and I were either getting married, graduating from college or moving to Massachusetts. She always had a logical reason for why we shouldn't get the dog. Now, we have a situation far more daunting than any we have faced in the past and she thinks that the timing is right to add a puppy to our lives.

"I can't wait either!" I fake a response, "I've been waiting for this day for a long time now, Jocelyn. It just seems kind of strange that we are rushing into this right now. You know given all that's happened."

"We aren't exactly rushing in, Matt. You've been talking about getting this dog since the day we met. When Zack passed away you had me in and out of every Phoenix area pet store looking at dogs. Now, we have found a little boy puppy, who doesn't shed and will be a perfect addition to our family."

I wish that I felt the same. A dog can last about fifteen years, given my diagnosis am I going to last another fifteen years? If so, will I be able to walk and care for this dog? I just wish someone had a crystal ball so I can see how this will all turn out.

We pull up to the kennel which is housed in a bright

yellow ranch. There is a statue of a dog and a small sign hanging which displays the kennel's name. Typically, Jocelyn would comment about the obnoxious color of the house, but today she is focused on getting inside to see the puppy.

There are small steps leading up to a breezeway. I slowly climb the steps as Jocelyn rings the bell. The door opens and I can hear the voice of a woman saying, "Can I help you?"

"Yes" says Jocelyn, "we are here to see the Wheaten puppies. My name is Jocelyn Cavallo. You took my deposit over the phone."

"Oh yes, Jocelyn. Come on in," the woman replies, "we've been expecting you. I'll run downstairs to get the litter."

Jocelyn enters the kennel and I follow behind her. The breezeway is an empty room. There is no furniture, just plain white walls with a door going to a basement and one to the main house. There are a couple of squeaky dog toys and a water bowl on the floor, making it evident that this is just a room to show puppies.

My hands are a sweaty and my heart is pounding faster. I can't believe that we are actually going to be getting a puppy in the next couple of minutes.

Moments later the door opens and the woman emerges carrying six puppies in a lined basket. She places the basket on the ground and out jump the puppies.

They start romping and stomping, wrestling and yelping, playing keep away with the toys. I can't help smiling an uncontrollable smile which I have been suppressing for months.

"They definitely have a lot of energy for eight weeks old," I say.

"They are a high energy breed," answers the woman, "even as adults Wheaten's typically keep their puppy enthusiasm.

As I watch all the puppies romp and play, there is one that stands out. Instead of playing with the rest of the puppies, this pup keeps following me around. This is not the biggest pup of the litter, so I assume it is one of the girls.

"Which one is the boy?" I ask.

"Couldn't tell you", the woman answers, "you'll just have to pick them up and look for yourself."

So, I chase the active puppies down, grabbing the biggest, which is also causing the most trouble. To my surprise, it is a female. So I grab the next biggest puppy and again it is a female. Meanwhile, this other puppy stays close to my feet, trying to nibble on my shoelace to get some attention. Finally, I pick up this puppy. This one wants me to pick it up and starts kissing my hands and face as I bring it close to me.

"You're a little lover," I whisper.

The tail is wagging profusely. Although the siblings are on the floor playing together, this one wants to be with me. Too bad you're going to be the girl, I think. No little boy could be this sweet.

"This one likes you a lot," Jocelyn says. "Do you think this is the one?"

"Probably not, Joci. We want the boy remember."

Then I turn the puppy over and to my surprise I can definitely tell that this is the boy after all! No mistake about it.

"I don't believe it Jocelyn! This is the boy. I think this is our puppy!"

She grabs me and hugs me and the puppy together. "Are we going to take him home?"

For the first time since getting this present, my anxiety melts. So what if I have MS, this puppy loves me for me. If somewhere down the road walking becomes an issue, I'm sure that he'll be ok. I have been beating myself up so badly over being diagnosed with a disease that I can't control that I have forgot that there is still so much to live for.

Jocelyn pays the lady the remaining balance and we are on the way home with a new member of the family. During the ride, the puppy sleeps on Jocelyn's lap. It is so natural, like he has always been with us.

"I can't believe it, Joci! Look at him. He loves you. You really found the perfect dog for us. What do you think we should call him?"

Jocelyn looks proudly down at our new puppy. "To me, he looks like a Teddy Bear. I think we should call him Teddy."

"I love it! Teddy it is!"

In this moment, I realize that everything is going to be ok. I have lost my legs for a period, but I didn't fully lose my will. The key is going to be to keep moving. I don't know how many steps I have left in these shoes, but I need to make all of them count.

As we pull into our driveway, I turn to Jocelyn and make a promise. "Jocelyn, no matter what is happening with my MS, I will make myself walk Teddy twice a day. No matter what."

I can see a tear form in her eye, but she holds it back, "Matt, I know you will and I will be there to help every step of the way. In fact, let's start now," she says with a wink, holding up Teddy's leash.

We get out of the car and start up the unevenly paved sidewalk of our neighborhood, following behind Teddy's puppy prance. Unsure of our path, but together. All three of us.

Chapter Thirty One - Life after Teddy

It has been seven years now since I was diagnosed with MS, and I have kept my promise. I walk Teddy each and every day. Once before work and once when I get home in the evening. While I have kept my promise, this is not to suggest that the past seven years have always been easy. In February of 2006, I came down with a case of Optic Neuritis and lost vision in my right eye for a period of time. During this time, I still managed to walk Teddy everyday while being treated with Solumedrol to regain my sight. In December of 2006, I started experiencing a cognitive loss similar to early onset Alzheimer's. I seemed to be forgetting everything, but each day I remembered to walk Teddy. I also became allergic to my once a week interferon treatment. Luckily, a new treatment called Tysabri re-entered the market. Some neurologists and patients were scared of the potentially fatal side effect that accompanied the drug but I decided to take a risk and started the treatment. I eventually had to have a cervical fusion operation to repair a fractured vertebra in September of 2010, which was related back to my Transverse Myelitis. This was a reminder that even though my symptoms are under control, the complications from MS can creep back into my life unexpectedly at anytime.

Today, I am thirty five years old, happy, healthy and feeling great overall. I am doing things today that I never dreamed about prior to being diagnosed with MS. Along with penning this memoir, I recently finished my Master's Degree in Public Health Informatics while training doctors, nurses and therapist on how to use medical software. I am the proud father of two beautiful boys, Mason and Colby, which I feared may not be possible when I was first diagnosed.

This may sound odd but being diagnosed with MS has

blessed my life in many ways. I have learned that "Yes, I am different and that is ok." I am more confident in my own skin and have a greater awareness of the world around me. I am not defined by my past, others' opinions of me, my material possessions, or my disease. I am Matt and that is good enough. For me the letters M and S now stand for My Strength. It is a strength that has been with me my whole life, although I didn't fully understand it until after I was diagnosed. It doesn't come from having a dog or an amazing career or even from having a perfect family. It comes from within ME and has allowed me to fight my MS as hard as I can to live the best life possible. The gift of learning to love and trust myself has allowed me to live each day not in fear of the future but in excitement about the new possibilities life has to offer.

I would like to share more with you about finding the power from within, but I have to go walk Teddy. Thank you for reading my story and best of luck on your journey.

Take care,

Matt

About the Author

Matt Cavallo is a passionate patient advocate who dedicates his life to the fight against Multiple Sclerosis. Matt has delivered motivational patient experience lectures all over the country for a variety of Multiple Sclerosis patient events. Matt has also appeared in a MS yoga DVD which is free for MS patients. Matt is active with MS charities and appeared in a documentary about the future of MS for the MS Cure Fund. Matt also worked for a Neuroscience Clinic, helping patients like himself every day. He recently finished his Master of Science in Health Care Informatics. Matt is also the proud father of Mason and Colby, the loving husband to his wife Jocelyn and the best friend of his dog, Teddy.

Connect with me Online

Personal Website: http://www.mattcavallo.com

Facebook: http://www.facebook.com/thedogstory

Twitter: http://twitter.com/#!/mattcavallo

Smashwords: http://www.smashwords.com/profile/view/mattcavallo

MS Yoga DVD: http://www.msactivesource.com/ms-yoga.xml

MS Cure Fund: http://www.mscurefund.org

Made in USA - Kendallville, IN
33418_9781477412992
03.16.2022 1434